Hot Topics in Acute Care Surgery and Trauma

Series Editors

Federico Coccolini
General Emergency and Trauma Surgery
Ospedale Bufalini
Cesena, Forli/Cesana, Italy

Raul Coimbra
Riverside University Health System – Medical Center
Riverside, CA, USA

Andrew W. Kirkpatrick
Dept of Surgery and Critical Care Medic
Foothills Medical Centre Dept of Surgery and Critical Care Medic
Calgary, AB, Canada

Salomone Di Saverio
Cambridge University Hospitals NHS Found
Department of Surgery (Addenbrooke)
Cambridge, Cambridgeshire, UK

Luca Ansaloni
Cesena, Italy

Zsolt Balogh
Newcastle, Australia

Walt Biffl
Denver, USA

Fausto Catena
Parma, Italy

Kimberly Davis
New Haven, USA

Paula Ferrada
Richmond, USA

Gustavo Fraga
Campinas, Brazil

Rao Ivatury
Richmond, USA

This series covers the most debated issues in acute care and trauma surgery, from perioperative management to organizational and health policy issues.
Since 2011, the founder members of the World Society of Emergency Surgery's (WSES) Acute Care and Trauma Surgeons group, who endorse the series, realized the need to provide more educational tools for young surgeons in training and for general physicians and other specialists new to this discipline: WSES is currently developing a systematic scientific and educational program founded on evidence-based medicine and objective experience. Covering the complex management of acute trauma and non-trauma surgical patients, this series makes a significant contribution to this program and is a valuable resource for both trainees and practitioners in acute care surgery.

More information about this series at http://www.springer.com/series/15718

Yoram Kluger • Federico Coccolini
Fausto Catena • Luca Ansaloni
Editors

WSES Handbook of Mass Casualties Incidents Management

Springer

Editors
Yoram Kluger
Department of General Surgery
Rambam Health Care Campus
Haifa
Israel

Federico Coccolini
General Surgery
Pope John 23 Hospital of Bergamo
Bergamo
Italy

Fausto Catena
Emergency Surgery Department
University of Parma
Parma
Italy

Luca Ansaloni
Surgery I
Pope John 23 Hospital of Bergamo
Bergamo
Italy

ISSN 2520-8284 ISSN 2520-8292 (electronic)
Hot Topics in Acute Care Surgery and Trauma
ISBN 978-3-319-92344-4 ISBN 978-3-319-92345-1 (eBook)
https://doi.org/10.1007/978-3-319-92345-1

This Springer imprint is published by the registered company Springer Nature Switzerland AG
The registered company address is: Gewerbestrasse 11, 6330 Cham, Switzerland

Preface

Mass casualty incidents (MCIs) as a result of man-made (accidental or not) or nature-induced mishaps inflict incredible stress even on the most experienced and knowledgeable system.

Numerous lives were saved in such events due to medical system preparedness. Whenever anticipatory readiness is not within an institutional objective, chaos will prevail.

Understanding the injury mechanisms and the resulting wounding potentials is important to combat influx of injured with compound injuries in an event of MCI, but this doesn't suffice.

The communal breaks in health system readiness around the world are well documented, and educational programs are often not addressed in a comprehensive and methodical manner. In many places around the world, mass casualty management plans and medical facilities preparedness plans are often developed and receive attention and response only after they have already experienced an MCI by themselves.

Conferring and sharing data with the experienced are the means of gaining understanding on the impact of MCI on the medical systems and the knowledge on how to cope with the major task of preparing a medical facility for a MCI wherever and anytime.

This book is a collection of some of the issues needed for the reader to initiate the process or to understand the prerequisites for MCI management. Indeed, the process should be started as previous and recent happenings indicate that MCI can occur in any place and at any time, even in the quietest part of the world.

Haifa, Israel Yoram Kluger

Contents

1 Mass Casualty Incident: Definitions and Current Reality 1
Laura Lomaglio, Luca Ansaloni, Fausto Catena, Massimo Sartelli, and Federico Coccolini

2 Managing a Medical Surge 11
Randy D. Kearns

3 Common Wounding Mechanisms and Injury Patterns 31
Miklosh Bala and Jeffry Kashuk

4 The Emergency Room During Mass Casualty Incidents 47
Hany Bahouth

5 Triage and Clinical Evaluation in MCI 61
Yoram Klein

6 Providing Information During Mass Casualty Incidents: Information Center, Family-Centered Care and Media Coverage 67
Roni Gagin, Neta HaGani, and David Ratner

7 Nurses and Nursing in Mass Casualties Incidents 79
Ben Rozenblit

8 Auxiliary Clinical Diagnostics 91
Miklosh Bala and Fausto Catena

9 Conventional and Interventional Radiology in Mass Casualty Incidents 101
Amos Ofer, Maxim Leiderman, and Nira Beck-Razi

10 Operating Room (OR) Setup, Resource, and Demands 117
Paola Fugazzola, Matteo Tomasoni, Yoram Kluger, Luca Ansaloni, and Federico Coccolini

11 Intensive Care Unit (ICU): Resources and Demands 121
Andrew J. Kamien, Christopher S. Davis, and Marc A. de Moya

12 The Pediatric Patient in MCI 129
Adam Lee Goldstein and Dror Soffer

13 Definitive Care Phase of a Mass Casualty Incident 143
Offir Ben-Ishay

14 Preparedness to Non-conventional Incidents in the Civilian Medical Arena 149
G. Shaked, D. Czeiger, and G. Sebbag

15 Mass Casualties Management in Low-Income Countries 157
Paola Fugazzola, Federico Coccolini, Cecilia Merli, Emiliano Gamberini, Vanni Agnoletti, and Luca Ansaloni

16 Mass Casualties Incident: Education, Simulation, and Training 167
Itamar Ashkenazi, Kristina Lennquist Montán, and Sten Lennquist

17 Debriefing Session: The Process of Self-Evaluation 177
Seema Yalamanchili, Sophie E. J. Hardy, and Christopher Aylwin

18 Ethics in Mass Casualty Incidents 189
Boris E. Sakakushev

Mass Casualty Incident: Definitions and Current Reality

1

Laura Lomaglio, Luca Ansaloni, Fausto Catena, Massimo Sartelli, and Federico Coccolini

1.1 Definitions of MCI and Related Concepts

The Pan American Health Organization (PAHO), which is the world's oldest international public health agency (N/A), defines a *Mass Casualty Incident* (MCI) "as an event which generates more patients at one time than locally available resources can manage using routine procedures. It requires exceptional emergency arrangements and additional or extraordinary assistance. For this reason, it can also be defined as any event resulting in a number of victims large enough to disrupt the normal course of emergency and health care services" [1].

These incidents are caused by a sudden and dramatic event, which can have a varying degree of severity depending on the place where it happens. For example, a bus crash in a small rural community with tens of injured survivors would fulfill the PAHO definition, as would a major natural disaster, such as a severe earthquake, affecting a heavily populated area. Both of these events can be considered MCIs, even if they pose very different challenges for the affected community and the emergency personnel that have to respond to them.

Before going on, some terms, with their related concepts, should be clarified.

A *hazard* is an event which has the potential to cause harm or loss. It may be natural or man-made.

L. Lomaglio (✉)
General Surgery Residency Program, University of Milan, Milan, Italy

L. Ansaloni · F. Coccolini
Unit of General and Emergency Surgery, Bufalini Hospital, AUSL Romagna, Cesena, Italy

F. Catena
Emergency Surgery Department, Parma University Hospital, Parma, OH, USA

M. Sartelli
General Surgery, Macerata Hospital, Macerata, Italy

Y. Kluger et al. (eds.), *WSES Handbook of Mass Casualties Incidents Management*, Hot Topics in Acute Care Surgery and Trauma,
https://doi.org/10.1007/978-3-319-92345-1_1

A *disaster* results from the interaction between a hazard and a community. This is a natural or man-made, sudden or progressive event, resulting in serious disruption of the functioning of the society, causing human, material, or environmental losses, exceeding the ability of the affected community to cope using its own resources. If a hazard impacts an isolated area, not affecting a community in any way, it will not cause a disaster [2].

The American College of Emergency Physicians (ACEP) focuses its attention on the health care resources when defining what a disaster is, stating that it occurs "when the destructive effects of natural or man-made forces overwhelm the ability of a given area or community to meet the demand for health care." Other definitions exist, but the common denominator is the inability of the organization, infrastructure, and resources of a community to return to normal operations without external assistance in the aftermath of the event [3].

The main features of a disaster are:

- Disasters interrupt the normal functioning of a community.
- Disasters exceed the coping mechanisms (capacity) of the community.
- External assistance is often needed to return to normal functioning of a community [2].

The *risk* is the probability of harmful consequences (expected loss of lives, injuries, property or environmental damage, disruptions in livelihood, and economic activity) resulting from a particular hazard for a given area in a certain period of time [2].

Vulnerability is the extent to which a community (with its structure, services, and environment) is likely to be damaged or disrupted by the impact of a hazard. For example, if a community has a high risk to be exposed to a flood, it can decrease or increase its vulnerability depending on the grade of preparedness that it develops. This is the reason why disasters do not occur every time a community is exposed to a hazard.

Vulnerability is therefore the combination of two factors: susceptibility and resilience. Susceptibility is the degree of exposure to a given risk (e.g., a community built by a river is more susceptible to floods than one built far from any watercourse is). Resilience is how well a community is able to face loss (e.g., a community that in the aftermath of a flood reconstructs safe houses with all facilities for its population in a small period of time is resilient).

To sum up, it is possible to express the relationship existing among risk, hazard, and vulnerability using the following formula: Risk = hazard × vulnerability [2].

1.2 Classification of Disasters, Levels of MCI, and Their Effects on Health and Hospitals

Disasters, and consequently the MCIs provoked by them, are generally classified into natural and technological (or human-made). However, in some situations, this distinction is not so neat, as there are frequent crossovers. Human actions can increase the risk of certain types of disasters (e.g., deforestation leading to landslides).

For these reasons, the most efficient system to manage an MCI would be an all-hazard approach, focusing on the level of MCI rather than on its causing event in order to be able to address both natural and man-made disasters.

1.2.1 Natural Disasters

Natural disasters can be classified as follows:

- Geophysical (earthquake, mass movement, volcanic activity, etc.)
- Hydrological (flood, landslide, wave action, etc.)
- Meteorological (storm, extreme temperature, fog, etc.)
- Climatological (drought, glacial lake outburst, wildfire, etc.)
- Biological (animal accident, epidemic, insect infestation, etc.)
- Extraterrestrial (impact, space weather, etc.) [4]

Tornadoes may be quite lethal but are generally short-lived. Hurricanes are more destructive than tornadoes; they tend to last longer and have more long-term recovery effects. They are, however, more predictable than other types of natural disasters thanks to modern technologies [5, 6].

Wildfires may persist for months and cause significant long-term damage. Volcanic eruptions can lead to a high number of fatalities but, as well as hurricanes, have become more predictable in recent years [2].

One of the most devastating natural phenomena are earthquakes. The number of deaths and injuries mainly depends on three factors: (1) building type/construction materials; (2) time of the day/night when the earthquake occurs; and (3) the population density of the area. Earthquakes tend to remain unpredictable, and populations have no time to evacuate or prepare for an impending event. In addition, local health care structures and hospitals can be largely affected. Specialized training and operation plans have been advocated to reduce morbidity and mortality in earthquake-prone regions [7].

Natural disasters may affect human health in many different ways. In fact, injuries and deaths occur directly not only from the event itself but also from its environmental consequences; malnutrition and increased morbidity and mortality from both communicable and non-communicable diseases (including mental diseases, e.g., posttraumatic stress disorder and psychological impairment) can be caused by malfunctioning in sanitation and reduced accessibility to health care [2].

Only advanced warning systems, structural and design improvements, and disaster planning may significantly decrease the devastation caused by many natural disasters. However, as populations occupy and develop areas that are at greater risk of specific types of natural disasters, the human and economic impact of these incidents keeps being likely to rise [3].

1.2.2 Technological (Man-Made) Disasters

Technological disasters tend to be more contained in terms of damages and losses than natural ones, but can also deliver a significant impact on life and property. Structural fires, toxic spills, and nuclear mishaps are included in this category of disasters, the first ones having caused some of the largest numbers of casualties in the USA.

In chemical, biological, radiological, or nuclear (CBRN) events, life or death is often determined within the first few minutes of their onset. For this reason, even before the detection and analysis of responsible agents can be undertaken, zoning, triage, decontamination, and treatment should be initiated as soon as possible [8].

Major transportation accidents, such as train derailments and airplane crashes, may quickly overwhelm the existing local emergency response system [3].

Other incidents having the potential to turn into mass casualties include war and terrorism, with bombings and blast injuries increasing in frequency with larger numbers of injuries and fatalities. Blasts also have the potential to involve radiological dispersion devices, the so-called dirty bombs. In these scenarios, chemical weapons have emerged as a serious potential threat, along with biological agents [3].

1.2.3 Levels of MCIs

MCIs are classified by levels, based on the number of potential victims generated by the causing incident. The emergency service response should be tailored and planned according to the level of the MCI:

- Level 1: 1–10 potential victims
- Level 2: 11–30 potential victims
- Level 3: 31–50 potential victims
- Level 4: 51–200 potential victims
- Level 5: More than 200 victims
- Level 6: Long-term operational period(s) [9]

Another way to classify MCIs is to consider the entity of the response—in terms of resources—required to face them:

- Level I MCI—requires local emergency response personnel and organizations to contain and deal effectively with the disaster and its aftermath.
- Level II MCI—requires regional efforts and mutual aid from surrounding communities.
- Level III MCI—is of such a magnitude that local and regional assets are overwhelmed, requiring national assistance.
- Level IV MCI—sometimes included in Level III; this MCI is of such magnitude that it requires international assistance and resources [2].

1.2.4 Direct and Indirect Impact of Disasters on Hospitals

A hospital/health care institution can directly be affected by a disaster when it is located in the impacted area, being damaged or destroyed. Hospitalized patients have limited mobility, so they are more vulnerable than the general population and may experience higher rates of morbidity and mortality; this must be taken into account when redacting an MCI management plan [2].

Indirect impact of disasters on hospitals occurs when they are located in the fringe of impact, triage, or organized aid area, as they will be inevitably called upon to play an important role in the response. In this case, hospitals may be asked to provide assistance in the form of manpower, materials supply, and logistics. Another aspect that has to be taken into account is that people from the local community may take shelter in the hospital [2].

During disasters, the points of care and the therapeutic strategies are completely different from the ones of "normal emergencies." This is well clarified in the following ACEP statement: "emergency medical services routinely direct maximal resources to a small number of individuals, while disaster medical services are designed to direct limited resources to the greatest number of individuals." This shift in priorities may represent a challenge for emergency services and physicians who are accustomed to dedicate all available resources to the most critical patients; damage control procedures may be more valuable than definitive diagnostics and treatments in these settings [3].

1.3 Epidemiology

According to historical data, the number of both natural and man-made recorded disasters has increased since 1900. The same has been registered as regards the number of victims [1].

According to the annual report of the Centre for Research on the Epidemiology of Disasters (CRED), in 2015, 346 disasters have been reported, the majority of which occurred in Asia (Fig. 1.1), with 22.773 million people dead and 98.6 million people affected (Fig. 1.2). The economic damage was estimated at 66.5 billion US dollars [4].

However, the MCIs that most countries experience more routinely are major accidents with tens of victims, rather than disasters with a larger number of victims. It will suffice to consider the example of September 11 attacks, which caused 2819 deaths; this number is only a small fraction of the 44,065 deaths from motor vehicle accidents occurred in the United States in 2002 [10]. Moreover, for each disaster listed in official disaster databases, about 20 other smaller emergencies with destructive impact on local communities are unacknowledged (Maskrey, cited in WHO 1999) [1].

As far as terrorism is concerned, some clarifications are needed. According to the fifth edition of the Global Terrorism Index (GTI), in 2016, there was a global decline

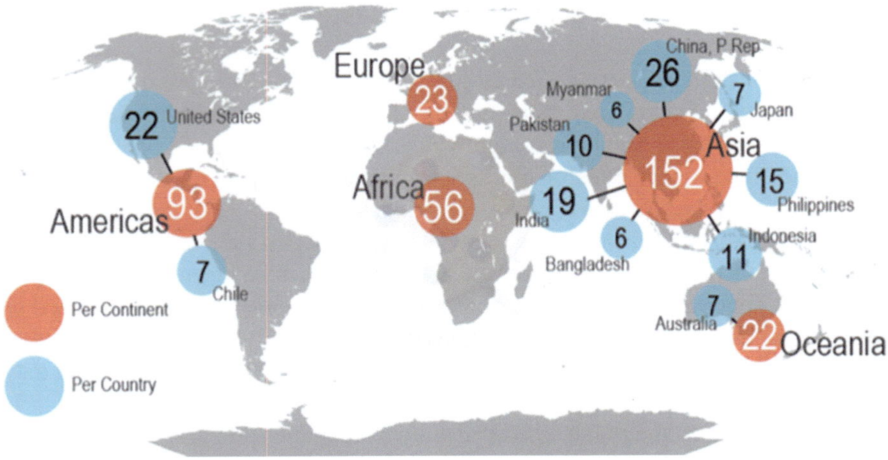

Fig. 1.1 Number of reported disasters per Country and Continent in 2015. The Countries indicated were the most affected. EM-DAT (25th January 2016): The OFDA/CRED—International Disaster Database www.emdat.be Université catholique de Louvain Brussels—Belgium

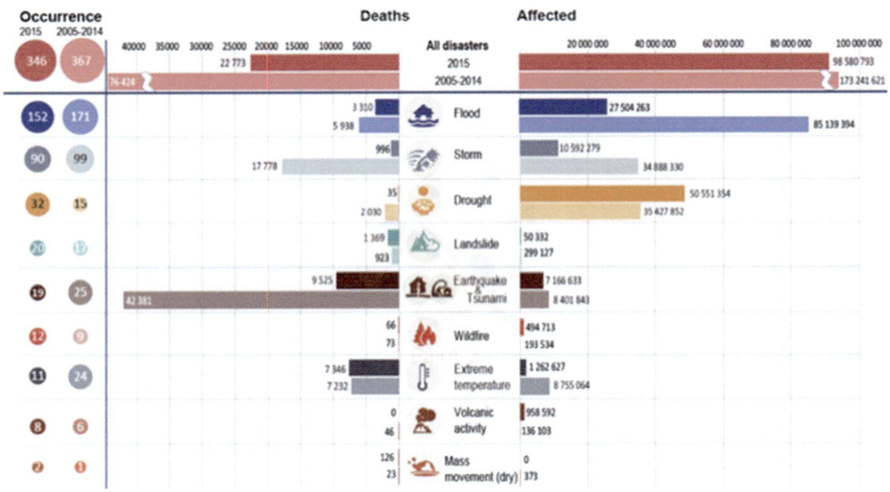

Fig. 1.2 Human impact by disaster types in terms of deaths and total people affected, comparing 2015 with the period 2005–2014. EM-DAT (25th January 2016): The OFDA/CRED—International Disaster Database www.emdat.be Université catholique de Louvain Brussels—Belgium

in the number of deaths from terrorism for the second successive year, with 25,673 people dead, which is a 22% improvement from the peak in 2014.

Over the last 15 years, South Asia experienced the majority of terrorist activity and the MENA region (Middle East and North Africa, N/A) had the sharpest increase in terrorism. The five countries most affected by terrorism are Iraq, Syria, Pakistan, Afghanistan, and Nigeria, which accounted for three quarters of all deaths from terrorism in 2016. It must be noted how, over the last 17 years, 99% of all terrorist deaths occurred in countries that are either in conflict or have high levels of political terror. Moreover, GTI shows how terrorist attacks are deadlier in conflict-affected countries (2.4 fatalities per attack in 2016 compared to 1.3 fatalities in non-conflict countries). This proves that the great majority of terrorism is used as a tactic within an armed conflict or against repressive political regimes. It also demonstrates the risks of political crackdowns and counterterrorism actions, which can exacerbate existing grievances and the drivers of extremism and terrorism.

In Organization for Economic Cooperation and Development (OECD, N/A) countries, there have been nearly 10,000 deaths from terrorism between 1970 and 2016, with 58% of these deaths occurred prior to 2000. ISIL is only the fourth most deadly terrorist group and accounts for 4.7% of terrorist deaths in OECD countries in the above-mentioned period of time. Separatist groups such as Irish separatists (IRA) and Basque nationalists (ETA) have killed over 2450 people since 1970, which is the 26% of the total deaths. OECD countries accounted for only 1% of global deaths from terrorism in 2016. This is, however, an increase from 0.1% in 2010 [11].

1.4 Principles of MCI Management

The range and unpredictability of where, when, and how events can occur, with all the possible variables that make each incident unique, including the number of victims, imply that planning and training to respond are extremely challenging. Preparedness is therefore the key to success in the effective management of an MCI, as endorsed by numerous resolutions passed by the World Health Assembly since 1981, when it first stated that "despite the undoubted importance of relief in emergencies, preventive measures, and preparedness are of fundamental importance." Preparedness implies consciousness that risk and vulnerability exist, and awareness by both government and local community of the benefit to plan and to have appropriate legislation.

In May 2007, the 60th World Health Assembly adopted a resolution that called, among other things, for WHO to provide guidance for the creation and strengthening of mass casualty management systems [1].

Despite these indications and the vast unfortunate experience of many countries around the world, preparedness toward MCI is not always institutionalized by proper management plans and health care personnel is not always sufficiently trained or updated, as showed for example by the World Society of Emergency Surgery (WSES) survey conducted in 2015 [12] and the report of the National Association of Emergency Medical Technicians (NAEMT) published in 2017 [13]. This outlines the paramount importance and the need to elaborate clear MCI management plans and promote courses—directed to all professionals involved in the response to an MCI, including health personnel—aimed to fill the gaps in MCI awareness and also to improve and optimize practical skills required in these exceptional situations.

An optimal MCI/disaster management should consider all four phases of the so-called disaster cycle: mitigation, planning, response, and recovery [3]. Paying particular attention on certain aspects of the cycle to the detriment of others may increase the harmful impact of events.

1. *Mitigation*: Some of the devastating effects of disasters can be reduced before the actual event. In this sense, useful measures are evacuations orchestrated before hurricanes and floods, as well as early forewarning from tornadoes and approaching hurricanes, in order for population to seek shelter; sprinkler systems in business and homes, to reduce the overall risk of total fire destruction; construction of anti-seismic buildings in earthquake prone regions.
2. *Planning*: In addition to be written, realistic disaster plans involve exercise, practice, and eventually revision, if found faulty or unworkable when applied. As an example, it must be considered that the initial search and rescue begin with victims and bystanders and not with trained rescue teams, and also the majority of patients arrive at hospitals without the intervention of the EMS system, so without having been triaged or decontaminated. Another important aspect to keep in mind when preparing a management plan is that it is impossible to plan for all contingencies: therefore, plans must be relatively general and expandable. Mutual aid agreements or contracts among existing area associations and institutions must be established before an actual event, in order to optimize the available resources as well as planning for funding and reimbursement.
3. *Response*: This phase of the disaster cycle tends to be considered the most important one, but an effective and coordinated response actually depends on the other three aspects of the disaster cycle. Response implies different aspects, which can be summarized as follows:
   - *Activation, notification, and initial response*: Organizations involved in disaster response and the potentially affected populations are notified.
   - *Organization of command and scene assessment*: Establishing a command structure is one of the most crucial steps to take once the disaster occurs. This must be prearranged and assembled almost immediately, as well as communication nets established. The Incident Command System (ICS) is an organizational and management tool used during disaster situations and emergency response operations (Fig. 1.3). Early assessment of the incident scene is also important to correctly prepare the arriving aid.
   - *Search and rescue*: Depending on the structure and function of the ICS, search and rescue may fall under the direction of fire, emergency medical services (EMS), police, or security forces. In large disasters, especially ones that are ongoing or that involve terrorist activities, a cooperative approach is necessary and the very act of search and rescue must be highly organized to ensure adequate and complete coverage of all areas.
   - *Extrication, triage, stabilization, and transport*: Extrication is performed by fire departments in most of the countries. Triage involves providing the most efficient aid to as many as possible and prioritizes treatment and transport of victims. Many variables influence the manner in which patients are triaged,

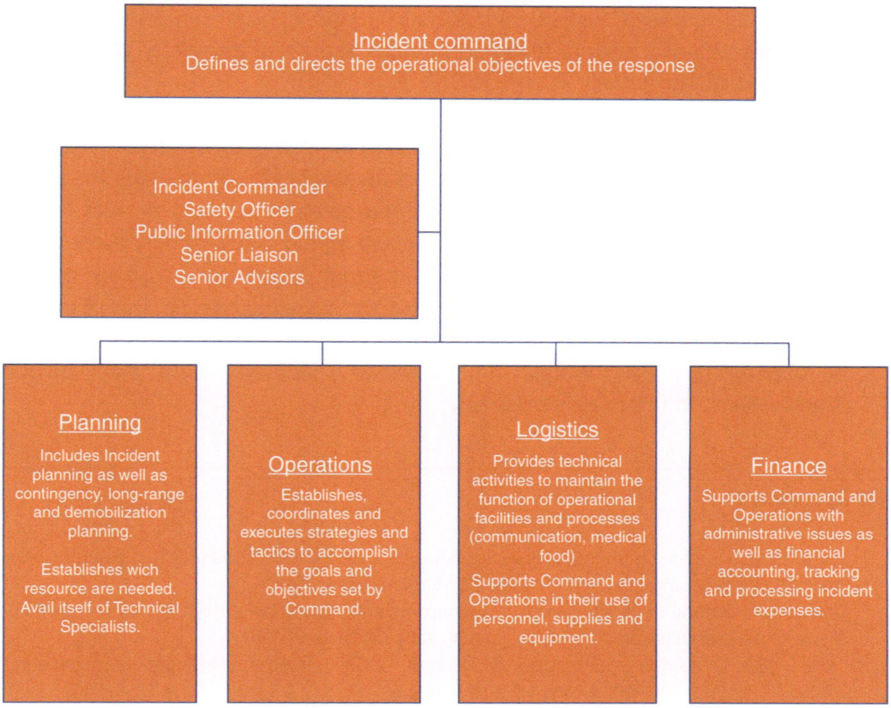

Fig. 1.3 The Incident Command System (ICS) model

transported, and treated: the type of incident, the number of victims, the available resources, the capability of existing infrastructure, and the overall context of the disaster. Patients must be reassessed during every step of the process. There are several algorithms for triage in mass casualty incidents that have been shown to have acceptable sensitivity and specificity in detecting severely injured patients [14, 15]. Errors in triaging may cause misallocation of valuable resources and may lead to worse outcomes among those affected. It is extremely important for health care providers to be familiar and trained in the triage system they are using. In some scenarios, such as extensive earthquakes, infrastructure may be damaged or destroyed to the extent that definitive care, even from outside resources, is not available for several days. In this case, dynamic treatment and recurrent triage of patients should be performed until other sources of medical care become available.

Transport must be both organized and orchestrated to equitably distribute victims to capable receiving facilities. Many of the less critically injured will self-extricate and arrive at the nearest medical facility by their own means. Often, the more critical patients arrive after the first wave of so-called walking wounded, and it is important to distribute these patients to appropriate receiving facilities with the capacity to take care of them. This process lessens the overwhelming impact a disaster may have on the closest hospital and improves the effectiveness of medical care provided to the victims. Victims may require decontamination prior to transport in order to prevent the spread of a hazardous material or threat.

– *Definitive scene management*

4. *Recovery*: This last phase is crucial for the affected community: order is restored, public utilities are reestablished, and infrastructure begins to operate effectively. Rebuilding and restructuring may include mitigation measures, in order to prevent or, at least, diminish the degree of damage in the case of a new event.

   Treatment of the responders is also important during this phase for critical stress debriefing. Debriefing may teach planners valuable lessons. It is of utmost importance to obtain as much information as possible from all parties involved in the disaster response. Without full disclosure, similar pitfalls may impede improvements in future responses [3].

References

1. World Health Organization. Mass casualty management systems. Strategies and guidelines for building health sector capacity. Geneva: The Organization; 2007.
2. Directorate General of Health Services, Government of the People's Republic of Bangladesh. A guide book on mass casualty management. Aalpoth Media; 2010.
3. Furin MA. Disaster planning. Medscape. 2016. https://emedicine.medscape.com/article/765495-overview. Updated 10 May 2016.
4. Guha-Sapir D, Hoyois P, Below R. Annual disaster statistical review 2015: the numbers and trends. Brussels: CRED; 2016.
5. Doocy S, Daniels A, Dooling S, Gorokhovich Y. The human impact of volcanoes: a historical review of events 1900-2009 and systematic literature review. PLoS Curr. 2013. https://doi.org/10.1371/currents.dis.841859091a706efebf8a30f4ed7a1901.
6. Doocy S, Dick A, Daniels A, Kirsch TD. The human impact of tropical cyclones: a historical review of events 1980-2009 and systematic literature review. PLoS Curr. 2013. https://doi.org/10.1371/currents.dis.2664354a5571512063ed29d25ffbce7.
7. Schultz CH, Koenig KL, Noji EK. A medical disaster response to reduce immediate mortality after an earthquake. N Engl J Med. 1996;334(7):43844.
8. Ramesh AC, Kumar S. Triage, monitoring, and treatment of mass casualty events involving chemical, biological, radiological, or nuclear agents. J Pharm Bioallied Sci. 2010;2(3):239–47.
9. Massachusetts Department of Public Health. The Massachusetts Emergency Medical Services (EMS) Mass Casualty Incident (MCI) Plan. 2016.
10. CDC. Deaths in world trade center terrorist attacks New York City, 2001. Morb Mortal Wkly Rep. 2002;51(Special Issue):1618.
11. Institute for Economics and Peace. Global terrorism index 2017: measuring and understanding the impact of terrorism. Sydney: Institute for Economics and Peace; 2017.
12. Ben-Ishay O, et al. Mass casualty incidents—time to engage. World J Emerg Surg. 2016;11:8.
13. Goodwin J. NAEMT National Survey on EMS preparedness for disaster and mass casualty incident response. 2017. http://www.naemt.org/docs/default-source/ems-agencies/EMS-Preparedness/2017-naemt-ems-preparedness-report.pdf?sfvrsn=0. Accessed X.
14. Benson M, Koenig KL, Schultz CH. Disaster triage: START, then SAVE—a new method of dynamic triage for victims of a catastrophic earthquake. Prehosp Disaster Med. 1996;11(2):11724.
15. Garner A, Lee A, Harrison K, Schultz CH. Comparative analysis of multiple casualty incident triage algorithms. Ann Emerg Med. 2001;38(5):5418.

Managing a Medical Surge

2

Randy D. Kearns

2.1 Introduction and History

Managing a surge of patients during a mass casualty or disease outbreak event has been described throughout history since healthcare began to be delivered in an organized manner. This includes the scope and scale of a given disaster, the quantity or quality of available resources, and the geopolitical implications of a particular event. Most historical accounts of mass casualty management are directly related to the battlefield. They involve medics and ambulance corpsmen at the point of conflict with military surgeons and other medical personnel just outside the battlefield.

Plagues and pandemics ravaged much of Europe between the fourteenth and eighteenth centuries, which spurred the evolution and better scientific understanding of medicine. The method that emerged as the best way to manage illnesses and reduce the spread of disease was to separate the sick patients (those with an infectious disease) from the general public. The infirmed patients were moved to buildings known as a pesthouse (lazaretto and quarantine station were synonymous terms as well) (Figs. 2.1 and 2.2).

Military medicine in the nineteenth century was limited to dressing and bandaging wounds, pharmaceutical comfort care, probing wounds for projectiles, and frequent amputation for extremity gunshot wounds. Near the battlefield, these surgeons and other medical personnel honed their training to deal with war-related injuries. If the arm or leg had a gunshot wound injury, surgeons became skilled in

R. D. Kearns (✉)
University of New Orleans, College of Business Administration, New Orleans, LA, USA

University of North Carolina, School of Medicine, Chapel Hill, NC, USA
e-mail: randy_kearns@med.unc.edu

Y. Kluger et al. (eds.), *WSES Handbook of Mass Casualties Incidents Management*, Hot Topics in Acute Care Surgery and Trauma,
https://doi.org/10.1007/978-3-319-92345-1_2

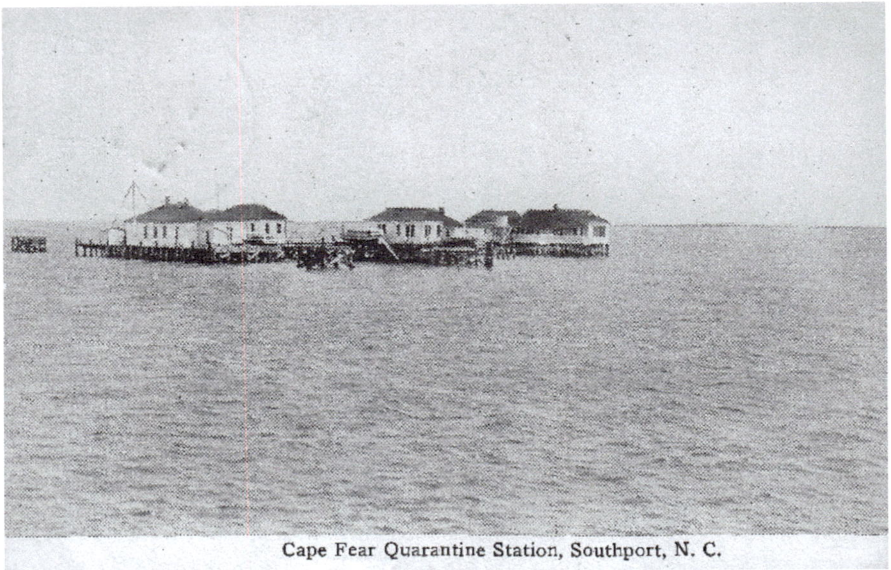

Fig. 2.1 Circa 1910 postcard from the author's personal collection. Many outbreaks of communicable disease overwhelmed port cities in the eighteenth, nineteenth, and early twentieth centuries. In an attempt to manage communicable disease patients, quarantine stations with hospitals or hospitals for mariners (generally known as Marine Hospitals) were built at ports to isolate and provide care for the sailors who were sick. Pictured in Fig. 2.1 is the Quarantine Station and Hospital Built on the Cape Fear River, the required entry point for Southport, North Carolina in the USA. Pictured in Fig. 2.2 is the US Marine Hospital built in Wilmington, North Carolina in the USA which opened in 1859

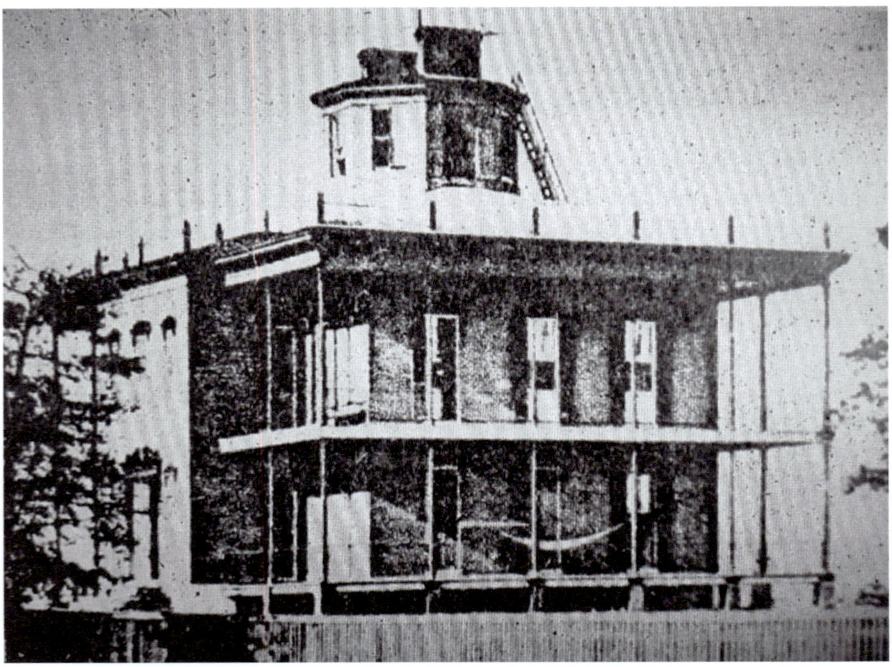

Fig. 2.2 Circa 1880 photograph from the New Hanover Public Library collection. Public Domain

quickly amputating the injured limb just above the wound. Prior to the discovery of antibiotics, this procedure was typically lifesaving since these injuries were commonly associated with death by infection.

During the nineteenth centuries, most civilian illness and injury continued to be managed in the home with doctors making house calls. The mass casualty incident was some calamity such as a passenger train crash, structure fire, or shipwreck. Patients were taken to large buildings such as hotels and boarding houses, with local doctors being summoned to aid the injured. When there was a civilian hospital, it was most likely near an ocean or river port and constructed there primarily for sick and injured sailors. These buildings were seldom more than what could best be described as a pesthouse or sanatorium for the patients with communicable diseases. There were few resources for mass casualty incidents.

2.2 Surge and the Lessons of War and Pandemic

The twentieth century witnessed two world wars, other multiple armed conflicts, and a global pandemic. Surgical medicine and infectious disease management were coming of age. Medical management during the Great World War of the early twentieth century included lessons learned from battlefield medicine following the Crimean and the American Civil Wars. Those lessons learned included a more orchestrated and deliberate management and movement of many patients relying on horse-drawn and motorized ambulance coaches, triage, and field surgical hospitals performing surgeries beyond the scope of extremity amputation [1].

As the Great World War commanded much of the global attention in 1918, a novel H1N1 influenza virus was quickly reaching pandemic status. The virus silently moved throughout much of the world's temperate climates killing millions of people [2]. Civilian hospitals were quickly overwhelmed by the surge of infirmed patients. As the numbers of patients swelled, so did the need to house these patients. Tent hospitals were erected, and public buildings were adapted to be used as temporary emergency hospitals [3]. Unlike much of the previous experiences with war and disaster, the pandemic virus struck many of the clinicians as well. As clinicians fell ill, the added struggle included managing the surge of patients with a depleted and frightened workforce (Fig. 2.3).

World War II, the Korean War, and other regional armed conflicts tested or drove innovations in ambulance evacuation, triage, and field hospitals. The Cold War fueled funding and expansion of civil defense programs internationally which included a medical surge component based on the threat of thermonuclear war [4].

As the Vietnam War raged, a glaring gap in trauma and ambulance care was being debated in the United States of America (USA) leading to improved trauma systems, an organized Emergency Medical Service (EMS) system both in the USA and internationally [5]. European trauma care and ambulance services were also rapidly evolving in the 1960s as well. By the early 1970s, these efforts to improve emergency care extended across much of the continents from Europe to Australia and North America.

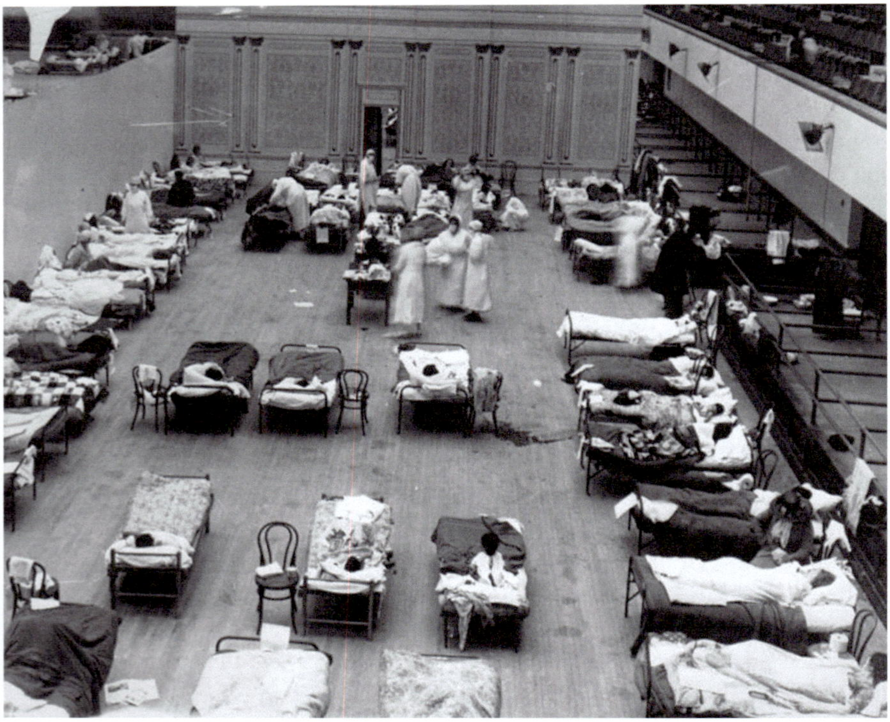

Fig. 2.3 Temporary Emergency Hospital erected in the Oakland Municipal Auditorium (California USA) in 1918 to manage the surge of patients during the influenza pandemic. The photograph depicts volunteer nurses from the American Red Cross tending influenza sufferers in the Oakland Auditorium, Oakland, California, during the influenza pandemic. Photo by Edward A. "Doc" Rogers. From the Joseph R. Knowland collection at the Oakland History Room, Oakland Public Library. Public Domain

2.3 The Twenty-First Century

In the aftermath of the 11 September 2001 (9/11) attacks, American and international disaster planners reexamined the various aspects of medical disaster planning and preparedness. Combining the 9/11 experiences with lessons learned from the international community and military planners who had dealt with mass casualty experiences involving a surge of patients during a disaster, a more coherent process began to emerge [6, 7].

2.4 The 2009 Influenza Pandemic

A 2005 threat of an H5N1 influenza pandemic did not emerge as many had feared [8]. Nevertheless, the anthrax attacks and 9/11 did influence the creation of a more coherent approach to surge focused on stratifying surge capacity and associating the escalating conditions with the standard of care [9]. Key components of this work were being refined about the same time as the 2009 H1N1 influenza pandemic.

While not as widespread or deadly as the 1918 H1N1 influenza pandemic, the surge of patients potentially needing a ventilator added to the importance of understanding capacity and capability when addressing surge needs. The potential ethical decisions were significant. Although there were sufficient space and personnel to manage the surge of patients, the shortfall focused on how many ventilators were available to include the circuits and personnel needed to keep them going. Critical questions that commonly arose included: how did the inventory match the potential influx of patients and if the patient numbers dramatically exceeded the capacity, what process was (or processes were) in place to decide who received the benefit of the ventilators? [10, 11]. Other areas of concern included the question of adequate policies and processes in place to aid in this decision-making process? While efforts were made to offer guidance for decision-makers in these grim ethical dilemmas, fortunately, those difficult decisions were typically not required and continue to be an ongoing source of concern across disciplines and continents [10, 12, 13].

Additional guidelines were published (2012) by Hick et al. [14] to further aid the clinicians with how to allocate scarce resources relying on a "planned, structured approach to include reactive and proactive triage guidelines" during a crisis surge capacity. The publication specifically identified six supply utilization strategies. They included "prepare, conserve, substitute, adapt, reuse, and reallocate." Furthermore, the triage focus of Hick et al. included objective assessments with a determination to not over-triage the patient population. The evidence continues to indicate a natural tendency to over-triage patients in an MCI.

2.5 Lessons Learned and Refined

At the onset of the disaster, there are three fundamental principles to be considered when managing a surge of patients. Those principles include rapid triage and moving patients to where they can best be managed for their specific injuries. In certain circumstances, it may also include deploying, redeploying, or moving equipment and personnel to where a large group (or groups) of patients are located. The overall strategy includes allocating resources in a manner that leverages and maximizes existing personnel, space, and equipment.

Disasters are local events, and community MCI planning is essential to attain optimal patient outcomes. Capacity and capability are inherently resource-based. This requires the development and implementation of thoughtful, carefully crafted, and individually designed emergency plans that match potential needs with a progressive echelon of available or potentially available response assets [15].

First-responder personnel commonly consist of local emergency medical services (EMS), fire, or rescue assets. However, training and available equipment often vary significantly between communities. Furthermore, the initial medical facilities that receive the first wave of patients may range from major regional tertiary medical centers to minimally staffed small community hospitals or clinics. This may include the use of temporary mobile hospitals in extraordinary situations [16, 17] (Fig. 2.4).

Given the known and anticipated variabilities in available resources, pre-incident planning is crucial. This planning contributes to the provision of consistent care delivered through the rational coordination of integrated system-level care networks [14, 18–20]. Unfortunately, there is ample evidence to suggest that this planning effort is not in an ideal state of readiness on many fronts [21–25]. When disaster strikes, the first call for help is typically routed to the local emergency communications center. (While there is no international consistency, the three most common emergency numbers include 1-1-2, 9-1-1, or 9-9-9.)

Once the call is placed to the emergency communications center, the trigger point for most disasters with a medical component flows through the local EMS system. Thus, the first wave of acutely injured or ill patients will be managed by EMS personnel (the *First Responders*) and the emergency department physicians and nurses and other hospital personnel (the *First Receivers*). Initial casualty evacuation may

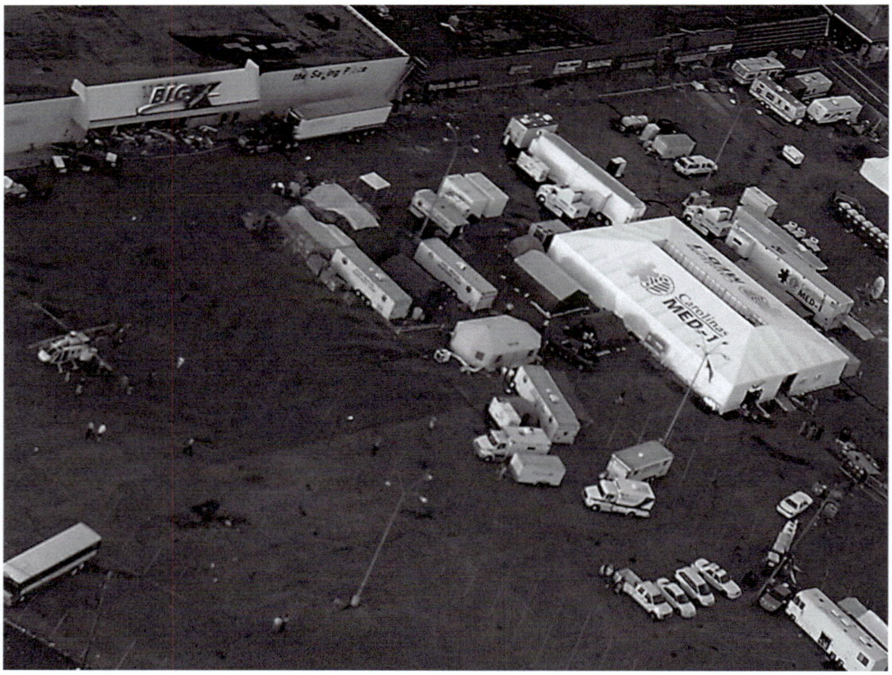

Fig. 2.4 A photograph of a mobile hospital (part mobile trailer unit and part tent) erected in the aftermath of Hurricane Katrina near Waveland, Mississippi USA August 2005. During the eight weeks of operation, the facility managed approximately 7500 patients and saw an additional 14,000 in need of vaccinations or replacement medication prescriptions. Along with approximately 100 staff, the hospital could manage 50–150 patients. Additional components can be added to hospitals such as this to substantially increase the bed capacity into the 400–600 patient range. (Photograph by the author)

include any available resource such as privately owned and other emergency service vehicles not typically designated for patient transport.

Provided there are multiple hospitals (first receivers) in the general area convenient to the site of the MCI, and sufficient planning is in place, a distribution of these patients from the scene can minimize the impact on the healthcare systems and potentially improve the outcomes [26, 27]. Otherwise, the closest hospital becomes the site where all patients are transported. This immediate surge of patients quickly becomes both a great challenge to manage the patients and a threat to keep the hospital or healthcare system operating without systems being overwhelmed during the disaster [14, 28]. Learning from these events, (whether civilian or military,) offers opportunities for improvement in an approach to MCI and overall surge management [29].

2.6 Capacity and Capability

Capacity refers to the quantity of staff, space, and supplies (pharmaceuticals and equipment) available. Capability refers to the types of clinicians available to render appropriate care for the sick and injured as well as the quality of equipment needed to perform certain procedures. The ability to manage one patient with a critical injury is not, by extension, an indication that large numbers can also be effectively managed by the same team of personnel without adequate expertise, planning and preparedness. Regardless, every medical facility should periodically review their operations to determine their capability as well as their capacity to manage a surge of patients during and following mass casualty event.

Key factors that determine capacity include commonly available resources in addition to critical assets that can be flexed to specifically accommodate MCI needs. The additional space needs can include holding areas, outpatient facilities, doubling the capacity of private hospital rooms, using conference rooms, and may include temporary structures as well [30, 31]. An important measure of scalable capacity is the ability to increase bed availability through flexing by 20% within 4 hours for the highest acuity patients [30].

Factors to consider in a capability analysis include available equipment and its asset typing, noninventory materials that have the potential for shipping and receiving, and available personnel with detailed credentialing information [20]. Also, an understanding of transportation assets including those that are local as well as those considered multijurisdictional, and multiagency is imperative [26, 32].

2.7 Facility Planning

Over the past 15 years, disaster planners and clinicians have gained a greater understanding of the assessment and management of mass casualty incidents with regard to the balance of **staff, space, and supplies** [33–35]. An emerging focus of surge included three defined categories: ***conventional, contingency, and crisis surge capacities*** [9, 32].

Depending on the event and the resources of the local facilities, smaller MCIs may be managed with minimal strain on existing healthcare resources. At times, surging requires only small modifications in staffing, hospital-based equipment, and treatment facility spaces. In these cases, traditional standards of care typically remain unchanged.

If the surge of patients overwhelm the resources of the local facilitie, traditional standards of care and expectations require modification. ***Contingency surge capacity (also known as contigency care)*** measures may include such things as provision of medical care in otherwise nontraditional settings or by nontraditional practitioners. Staffing will typically include clinicians with traditional credentials but who may be unaccustomed to the specialized care that will need to be delivered. Supplies are commonly limited in these settings, and in some cases, substitute medications or fluids may need to be used. The most unpredictable limitation is the availability of and access to supplies and specialty equipment such as intravenous pumps and ventilators.

Crisis surge capacity (also known as crisis care) implies that the practices of care may, by necessity, extend outside of what is considered traditional standards of care. Although often required under these conditions, mitigation strategies should be enacted to alleviate them as soon as reasonably possible. The pre-incident planning process provides an ideal opportunity to engage informed policymakers [12, 13, 18]. This process should include standards under various potential disaster scenarios, provide guidelines for acceptable care under resource-constrained conditions, and outline reasonable expectations for the infrastructure needed to manage disaster event. Depending on the nature, size and scope of the event, crisis care could continue for days, weeks or months for several of the more devistating disaster scenarios (such as the 2004 Tsunami in Banda Aceh, Indonesia or the 2010 Earthquake in Port-au-Prince, Haiti.) The most important step in managing a surge of patients starts with planning for a surge of patients.

2.8 Surge Equilibrium

As a disaster scenario unfolds, there are trigger points that often mark event stabilization. The achievement of this state of relative balance (known as ***surge equilibrium***, represented in Fig. 2.5) can be identified when sufficient numbers of patients (which includes those who have been transferred, discharged, or died) and their ongoing needs can be met on a steady and predictable basis by the staff, space, and supplies available for use. Effective and efficient transportation resources are practical tools to enable relative patient decompression during a disaster by both allowing rational triage of acutely injured or ill patients to appropriate receiving facilities and simultaneously shuttling supplies, personnel, and (if needed) temporary treatment facilities to the disaster site.

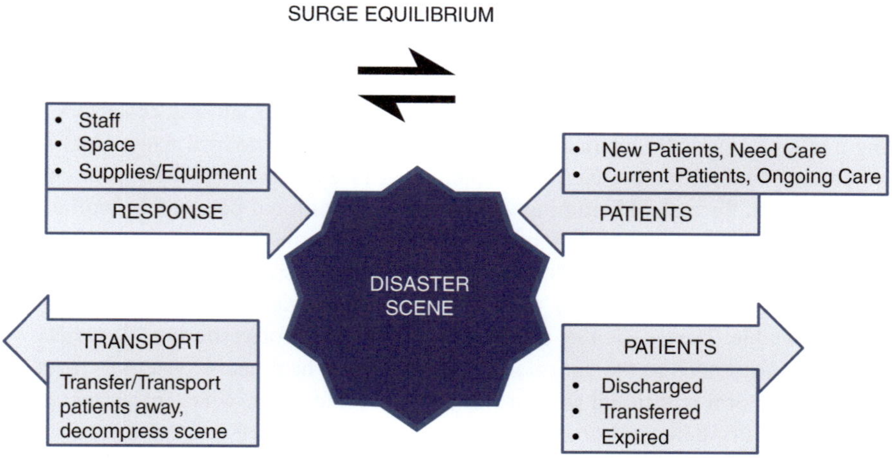

Fig. 2.5 Surge equilibrium: all competing influences of the disaster are balanced at the point of where the patients are being managed, at the disaster scene, or at a medical facility such as the hospital or clinic. (Image and concept created by the author)

2.9 Immediate Bed Availability

A core strategy for disaster process planning is the implementation of an Immediate Bed Availability (IBA) approach. This solution emphasizes the deliberate reverse triage and discharge of affected patients to make available medical resources with reliance on existing personnel to receive and treat the initial influx of patients from an MCI. It is believed that reasonable IBA tactics can generate 20% additional resources with no more than a 4-hour notice [30].

2.10 Just-in-Time Training, Alternative Staff Resources, and Force Multipliers

Strategies to increase staff include force multipliers through just-in-time (JIT) training by utilizing personnel who have the aptitude to quickly learn, adapt, and assist [36]. Cross-training before a disaster can augment personnel pools in preparation for an MCI event, but logistically may not be a viable option for smaller organizations. Military surge strategies offer excellent examples of how to systematically leverage medical resources by flexing available workforce that may not be considered traditional clinical complements. JIT training paradigms can augment targeted capabilities over relatively short timeframes and can provide large groups of caregivers lead by specially trained medical team leaders, allowing systems to manage large numbers of acute care patients [37, 38].

Telemedicine platforms may also be used to augment staff and provide expert assistance "virtually" when the necessary technology is available to support the effort [39].

Effective strategies that are commonly used to expand staffing resources during a crisis surge is the planned incorporation of disaster medical responders from other communities via preexisting memoranda of understandings (MOU) or capacity expansion through JIT training and use of nontraditional personnel. Availability of these resources varies widely between jurisdictions and home countries. Ideally, additional support could include government disaster resources [40].

The inherent complexity of disasters that include varied types of trauma and communicable disease creates a potential competition for resources. A variety of patient injuries adds to the enormous pressure on the healthcare system to meet all of the needs of a traditional standard of care [41]. However, when infrastructure is catastrophically damaged or destroyed (e.g., earthquakes or war), the result may include a crisis standard of care dominating the immediate care environment for potentially an extended period of time. The downstream effect includes extending the stress into a region well beyond the impacted area. As such, earthquakes or any natural or man-made disaster that creates widespread damage to the infrastructure must be considered in the disaster planning efforts [41].

2.11 Three Stages of Activity During a Surge Plan and One Consideration

Disaster planning should include a surge component. This may take the shape of an annex to a multihazard plan or a standalone plan for surge. Regardless, critical components of a surge plan, or a disaster plan for that matter, should address these objectives.

2.11.1 Stage 1: Activation Point/Trigger(s)

Disaster plans must include an activation point (trigger). Triggers are identified by a combination of data or science and the opinions of the subject matter experts. All disaster plans should offer sufficient latitude to move into the context of the plan early on in the disaster, in an attempt to maintain stability and avoid the tendency toward chaos.

2.11.2 Stage 2: Functional Period of Activity

Disaster plans must have a functional period of activity. This functional activity can be tested and assessed through a variety of methods. Simulation provides an opportunity to simultaneously test numerous inputs and variables in a cost-effective lab setting, to identify potential plan weaknesses and augment plan strengths [42–45].

Three commonly employed modeling techniques include Monte Carlo Simulation, Discrete Event Simulation, and Continuous Simulation. Modeling is routinely performed in an academic environment, and numerous published surge models exist based on these systems [45–53].

Methods to test planning efforts can include (virtual) table-top exercises, functional scenarios (where one or more specific components are tested), and full-scale simulation involving the physical participation of many personnel and structures [54]. In the aftermath of any disaster, it is essential to develop an after action report (AAR) to identify successes as well as opportunities for improvement, where existing plans can be modified or improved based on actual experiences. Incorporating Lean and Six Sigma tools, such as spaghetti plots and process maps, can significantly enhance the quality of AARs.

2.11.3 Stage 3: Event Termination

All surge events have a conclusion. It is important to mark that conclusion and plan for the demobilization of resources and personnel specifically assigned to the disaster. Returning to a state of normalcy is essential both functionally for the institution and mentally for personnel. Aside from pandemics, certain disasters (earthquake, cyclones, hurricanes, landslides) have a prolonged operational period such as when infrastructure has been damaged, and there may be an extended period of search and rescue.

2.11.4 Consideration: Plan Failure

No disaster plan is infinitely scalable and can address all possible scenarios. When the plan attempts to address a range from the common to the more obscure of potential disaster scenarios, the resulting document can become unwieldy and potentially less effective. A surge plan should stay focused and include critical elements, common scenarios, and key indicators which can be tracked and measured during and following the event.

There are rare or unforeseen situations where a plan could fail to keep the patient surge contained by the efforts of the plan such as an earthquake that damages much of the hospital or the detonation of an improvised nuclear device. Both scenarios are unlikely but should either occur; key elements of any surge plan will include framework elements for addressing the surge. These elements include augmenting the workforce, using ancillary space for additional patients, and securing all available supplies until patients can be treated and released or treated and transferred away from where the surge has occured or resources and personnel moved into the scene or at the facility.

Any plan must also consider where additional resources can be accessed and facilitate efficient and effective coordination with other hospitals or tertiary medical centers within an immediate area (referred to as interfaculty planning). Based on geography and proximity, the closest resources may be in a different jurisdiction or country and should be reflected in the plan.

2.12 Initial Keys to Create a Surge Plan

A basic surge plan starts with these two questions:

- What information is available or can easily be accessed to identify known hazards and what is the potential patient count? [Two of the more common approaches to a hazard identification and vulnerability analysis include the Hazard Vulnerability Analysis (HVA) and the Threat and Hazard Identification and Risk Assessment (THIRA)].
- What are the resources available to manage the surge of patients? (Table 2.1)

Table 2.1 Surge plan: key questions and considerations

Purpose: Creating a surge plan starts with reviewing the potential threat(s) or hazard(s) using the process of threats, hazard identification and risk assessment (THIRA), or hazard and vulnerability analysis (HVA). This assessment focuses on events that could produce a surge of patients while considering existing resources as well as those which could reasonably be anticipated. The plan starts with identifying "triggers" or activation points that set into motion, the use of the surge plan.
Surge plan options: A surge plan should be a component of the larger planning process for an organization. This larger planning process typically starts with the emergency operations plan (EOP) (base plan), be an addendum to the EOP, or may include a series of annexes, appendices, or policies, procedures, and protocols also attached to the EOP. Many of the elements that should be addressed in developing a surge plan may already exist in the EOP, or other plans, policies, procedures, or protocols.
Surge plans (policies and procedures) should address internal and external communication regarding current emergency status for surge levels, the type, scope, expected duration of an event, and escalation/de-escalation as new information is received. The strength of a good plan includes "triggers," meaning adequate detail to allow implementation by staff who may not be familiar with the details of the plan. Job action sheets, field operation guides, task checklists, or other tools for activating and operationalizing the surge plan should be developed for this purpose.
It is presumed that general areas such as security, alternate care sites, command and coordination, and other ancillary and support services are outlined in the EOP. This tool is designed to aid the institutional medical surge plan due to the uniqueness and resource demand of a surge event.
This checklist should be used as one of several tools for evaluating your current surge plan or to aid in developing one. The plan should be developed in coordination with other related disaster plans. The surge plan should be consistent with your agency or hospital (organization's) emergency management procedures and policy for disaster response. Where applicable, all planning efforts should ensure compliance with governmental regulations and accreditation standards. Additional online resources to assist in surge and surge planning and with specific items are listed at the end of this document.

Table 2.1 (continued)

Status*	Plan elements
	The plan identifies triggers and decision-making processes for a surge event.
	Initial assessment of the event type, scope, and magnitude, the estimated influx of patients, the real or potential impact on the responding agency or receiving facility and special response needs.
	Notification of appropriate points of contact outside the agency initially involved (e.g., EMS, hospital, and public health). The agency or hospital EOP should identify all related contacts.
	Internal notification/communications and staff call-back protocols (call trees, contact information, etc.). Ensure a higher priority system is created for those who are most critical to the operation.
	Where applicable, establish ongoing communications with a regional coordination center. This activity could play a role in patient placement, resource distribution, or mutual aid response.
	Activation of resource management system including inventory, tracking, prioritizing, procuring, and allocating of resources. Event-specific supplies should be anticipated as the event unfolds and requested based on the EOP. (What do you have [internally] and who has a cache of supplies you can access if needed? [externally])
Immediate response: (Inventory) What are your available resources as a first responder? (Who can come to the scene to assist?) What are your resources as a first receiver or as the regional receiving facility? Who can receive patients from the scene or being transferred? The initial distribution of patients can ease surge needs with appropriate triage and destination choices early into the disaster.	
	Triage: Plan to activate and operate additional/alternate triage area(s) during a surge event. The activation of triage, as well as additional sites, should be outlined in the surge plan. The triage component of the surge plan should be followed with the following related changes: *Assumption: Triage area activation and operations are outlined in the surge plan.*
	• Development of activation triggers for establishing alternate/additional triage areas should be defined and exercised. The number of patients required to meet the threshold of a surge event will depend on the quantity of patients and their criticality. A small number of critical patients can quickly exceed the capability due to the complexity of care, supply needs, and personnel demand. The threshold of a surge event will also vary based on the conventional capacity and capability of a facility. Large, tertiary hospitals may routinely see large volumes and thus better prepared for larger numbers of sick or injured patients.
	• A functioning triage plan is essential for any agency/hospital involved in patient care. This plan (or policy/procedure) will be an important aspect of the surge plan and should be referenced in the surge plan.
	Decontamination: Plan to activate and perform decontamination, as necessary. • Ensure that the surge plan/EOP contains a means to address the need to separate and decontaminate (as indicated) patients during a surge event.
	Holding areas: Plan for activation and operation of holding areas for patients awaiting further triage, decontamination, treatment, admission, or transfer. • Ensure that the surge plan/EOP contains a means to address the need for holding areas.
	Treatment areas: Plan for activation and operation of additional treatment areas. • Ensure that the surge plan/EOP contains a means to address the need for treatment areas.

(continued)

Table 2.1 (continued)

Status*	Plan elements
	Security—facility access: Plan(s) for securing and limiting facility access during a surge event. • Ensure that the surge plan/EOP addresses the need for security.
Direct patient care areas	
	The function of communication and coordination regarding local community resources, regional, or state resources to expand patient care areas must be identified (e.g., a mobile field hospital). • Typically coordinated by the facility or organizational emergency management designee, will be included in the EOP.
	Potential conventional surge areas, contingency surge areas, and crisis surge areas are identified, the plan addresses alternate care facility/facilities, alternative care locations such as parking lots, and resources needed to set up field medical aid stations or temporary hospitals.
	Equipment resources or adaptations identified (inventory lists) including supplies with appropriate supplies in stock.
	Protocols for patient transfer to a facility with appropriate capabilities, when they become available.
Transportation	
	Depending on the agency or hospital involved the surge plan may include getting vehicles to the scene to move patients away from the scene (preferably their ideal destination with the first transport). This includes coordination with first responders (EMS agencies) and (first receivers) receiving facility (facilities) or for those being transferred from one hospital to another.
	Transportation considerations must address capabilities and constraints (e.g., geography, weather, and resources).
	Includes mutual aid transportation resources either specific to emergency care (ambulances, ambu-bus, critical care transport, and aeromedical resources) or more general resources such as buses. Also, include regional/state/federal assets such as ambulance strike teams.
Staffing	
	Specific plans for staffing during a significant surge event using hospital staff, contracted pools, and mutual aid resources, taking into consideration the type and scope of the event.
	• Identification of staffing needs by staff type and service area that should be prioritized during a surge event.
	• Staff disaster response assignments/roles (labor pool, specific units/areas, etc.) considering the type of event for personnel within the organization.
	• Protocols for requesting and receiving staff resources from outside the agency/hospital (volunteers, special needs/teams, etc.). This should include personnel registered through ESAR-VHP or other voluntary healthcare registry databases.
	• Cross-training and reassignment of staff to support critical/essential services.
	• Pre-establish just-in-time (JIT) training for key areas.
	• Protocols and specific assignment of appropriately trained professionals to monitor and assess staff for both stress-related and physical health concerns.
	Behavioral health needs: The plan addresses or references in the organization's EOP how behavioral health needs of staff, patients, and family members will be met. A surge event can be devastating for staff. The patient and family needs may be amplified in a surge event due to the magnitude, unsightliness, and devastation of the injuries.

Table 2.1 (continued)

Status*	Plan elements
	Care requirements for services not normally provided: The plan addresses protocols and resources for providing services to the injured patients which are not normally provided by the hospital.
Communications	
	Documentation—patient tracking: Minimum patient care documentation is required to assure an orderly flow and to account for all patients (this is typically addressed in a triage plan).
	With staff: The plan describes primary and backup external communication systems for contact with the local center or the coordination center or references how it is addressed in the organization's EOP.
	With media: A policy for media coordination is addressed in the organization's EOP. Dissemination of information should follow already established pathways.

Note the status of plan elements in the Status* columns (*C* completed, Pxx% noting the numerical value of percent progressing to completion, *NA* not applicable)

Hospital Incident Command System (HICS) resource websites: http://www.emsa.ca.gov/hics/

** Alternate Care Sites: https://asprtracie.hhs.gov/technical-resources/48/alternate-care-sites-including-shelter-medical-care/47

The Joint Commission, Emergency Management Chapter is available for purchase at: http://www.jointcommission.org/standards_information/standards.aspx

The California Hospital Preparedness website: http://www.calhospitalprepare.org

National Incident Management System (NIMS) (free) training: https://www.fema.gov/nims-training

CHA Hospital Surge Planning Resources: http://www.calhospitalprepare.org/category/content-area/planning-topics/healthcare-surge

Crisis Standards of Care: A Toolkit for Indicators and Triggers. Hanfling D, Hick JL, Stroud C. National Academies of Science. https://www.ncbi.nlm.nih.gov/books/NBK202381/

ESAR VHP: https://www.phe.gov/esarvhp/Pages/default.aspx

** Alternative care locations and alternate care sites were not originally synonymous but now tend to be interchanged. An example of a legacy use of an alternative care location is an urgent care or doctors office in lieu of a hospital, and alternate care sites were predetermined ranging from the adjacent office building to a hospital for a surge of patients or in preparation of large numbers of infected patients such as Avian Flu Pandemic or a Chem-Bio attack. The literature today indicates these terms are now (generally) interchanged.

*** This checklist originally began as an adaptation of the 2011 version of the California Hospital Association Surge Plan Checklist, and Resources Guide.

2.13 Discussion

Managing a surge of patients during a disaster requires planning, speed, repetition, training, and simplicity. Disaster plans should build upon daily and preplanned activities. If the use of triage tags is advocated and identified in a plan but used only during a mass casualty incident, the lack of familiarity can lead to failure. If response spaces and supplies for the surge of patients are never identified, and the staff is not trained to manage the surge, success, when this disaster strikes, is unlikely.

Clinicians are accustomed to managing patients based on the traditional standard of care. However, can they recognize the signs that response resources are being overwhelmed by patient needs during an ever-escalating event? When this happens, what is the plan and what are the processes to maintain control of the incident?

When disaster strikes, EMS is typically the first source of information and the first to start the process of managing the surge of patients. As the disaster unfolds, this will transition to the emergency department clinicians who will see the first wave of patients to include those patients who self-evacuate as well as those transported by EMS.

Conclusion

Recent events continue to underscore the importance of planning for a surge of patients with complex needs. The modeling, planning, and after action of real events should also identify potential failure points and who to call for assistance before being overwhelmed. Planning and preparedness activities by first responders, first receivers, and all involved leaders will minimize the confusion and needless loss of life and maximize the response to the disaster to include the allocation of resources. Creativity and luck can contribute to a successful outcome. However, they are weak substitutions for preparedness and planning activities long before the disaster ever occurs.

References

1. Simpson AT. Transporting Lazarus: physicians, the state, and the creation of the modern paramedic and ambulance, 1955-73. J Hist Med Allied Sci. 2013;68(2):163–97.
2. Murray CJ, Lopez AD, Chin B, Feehan D, Hill KH. Estimation of potential global pandemic influenza mortality on the basis of vital registry data from the 1918-20 pandemic: a quantitative analysis. Lancet. 2006;368(9554):2211–8.
3. Stern AM, Cetron MS, Markel H. The 1918-1919 influenza pandemic in the United States: lessons learned and challenges exposed. Public Health Rep. 2010;125(Suppl 3):6–8.
4. Dodge AH. The 1962 civil defense emergency hospital program. N Y State J Med. 1963;63:3144–6.
5. National Academy of Sciences (US) and National Research Council (US) Committee on Trauma, National Academy of Sciences (US) and National Research Council (US) Committee on Shock. Accidental death and disability: the neglected disease of modern society. Washington, DC: National Academies Press (US); 1966. https://doi.org/10.17226/9978. https://www.ncbi.nlm.nih.gov/books/NBK222962/.
6. Peleg K, Michaelson M, Shapira SC, Aharonson-Daniel L. Principles of emergency management in disasters. Adv Ren Replace Ther. 2003;10(2):117–21.
7. Rasmussen TE, Baer DG, Goolsby C. The giving back: battlefield lesson to national preparedness. J Trauma Acute Care Surg. 2016;80(1):166–7.
8. Alcock J, Delieu J. Planning for pandemic influenza. Nursing Standard (Royal College of Nursing (Great Britain): 1987). 2007;22(3):35–9.
9. Hick JL, Barbera JA, Kelen GD. Refining surge capacity: conventional, contingency, and crisis capacity. Disaster Med Public Health Prep. 2009;3(2 Suppl):S59–67.
10. White DB. Who should receive life support during a public health emergency? Using ethical principles to improve allocation decisions. Ann Intern Med. 2009;150(2):132.

11. Rubinson L, Hick JL, Curtis JR, et al. Definitive care for the critically ill during a disaster: medical resources for surge capacity: from a Task Force for Mass Critical Care summit meeting, January 26-27, 2007, Chicago, IL. Chest. 2008;133(5 Suppl):32S–50S.
12. Cusack L, Gebbie K. Call for national dialogue: adapting standards of care in extreme events. We are not ready. Collegian. 2017;24(1):93–100.
13. Leider JP, DeBruin D, Reynolds N, Koch A, Seaberg J. Ethical guidance for disaster response, specifically around crisis standards of care: a systematic review. Am J Public Health. 2017;107(9):e1–9.
14. Hick JL, Hanfling D, Cantrill SV. Allocating scarce resources in disasters: emergency department principles. Ann Emerg Med. 2012;59(3):177–87.
15. Healthcare Preparedness Capabilties, National Guidance for Healthcare System Preparedness. In: Response OotASfPa, editor. http://www.phe.gov/Preparedness/planning/hpp/reports/Documents/capabilities.pdf. US DHHS ASPR; 2012. p. 72.
16. Kearns RD, Stringer L, Craig J, et al. Relying on the National Mobile Disaster Hospital as a business continuity strategy in the aftermath of a tornado: the Louisville experience. J Bus Contin Emer Plan. 2017;10(3):230–48.
17. Blackwell T, Bosse M. Use of an innovative design mobile hospital in the medical response to Hurricane Katrina. Ann Emerg Med. 2007;49(5):580–8.
18. Adini B, Israeli A, Bodas M, Peleg K. Increasing perceived emergency preparedness by participatory policy-making (think-tanks). Disaster Med Public Health Prep. 2018;1–6.
19. VandenBerg SL, Davidson SB. Preparation for mass casualty incidents. Crit Care Nurs Clin North Am. 2015;27(2):157–66.
20. Kearns RD, Cairns BA, Cairns CB. Surge capacity and capability. A review of the history and where the science is today regarding surge capacity during a mass casualty disaster. Front Public Health. 2014;2:29.
21. Hashikawa M, Gold KJ. Disaster preparedness in primary care: ready or not? Disaster Med Public Health Prep. 2018;12(5):644–8.
22. Ortu G, Mounier-Jack S, Coker R. Pandemic influenza preparedness in Africa is a profound challenge for an already distressed region: analysis of national preparedness plans. Health Policy Plan. 2008;23(3):161–9.
23. Hodge JG Jr, Gostin LO, Parmet WE, Nuzzo JB, Phelan A. Federal powers to control communicable conditions: call for reforms to assure national preparedness and promote global security. Health Secur. 2017;15(1):123–6.
24. Eastman AL, Fabbri W, Brinsfield K, Jacobs L. Improving national preparedness for intentional mass casualty events: a seamless system of evidence-based care. J Trauma Acute Care Surg. 2016;81(5 Suppl 2 Proceedings of the 2015 Military Health System Research Symposium):S77–80.
25. Cordova-Villalobos JA, Macias AE, Hernandez-Avila M, et al. The 2009 pandemic in Mexico: experience and lessons regarding national preparedness policies for seasonal and epidemic influenza. Gac Med Mex. 2017;153(1):102–10.
26. Hall TN, McDonald A, Peleg K. Identifying factors that may influence decision-making related to the distribution of patients during a mass casualty incident. Disaster Med Public Health Prep. 2018;12(1):101–8.
27. Adini B, Bodas M, Nilsson H, Peleg K. Policies for managing emergency medical services in mass casualty incidents. Injury. 2017;48(9):1878–83.
28. Hick JL, Einav S, Hanfling D, et al. Surge capacity principles: care of the critically ill and injured during pandemics and disasters: CHEST consensus statement. Chest. 2014;146(4 Suppl):e1S–e16S.
29. National Academies of Sciences, Engineering, and Medicine. A national trauma care system: integrating military and civilian trauma systems to achieve zero preventable deaths after injury. Washington, DC: The National Academies Press; 2016.

30. Public Health Emergency. Immediate bed availability. 2014. http://www.phe.gov/Preparedness/planning/sharper/Pages/iba.aspx. Accessed 7 July 2016.
31. Kearns RD, Skarote MB, Peterson J, et al. Deployable, portable, and temporary hospitals; one state's experiences through the years. Am J Disaster Med. 2014;9(3):195–210.
32. Kearns RD, Hubble MW, Holmes JH 4th, Cairns BA. Disaster planning: transportation resources and considerations for managing a burn disaster. J Burn Care Res. 2014;35(1):e21–32.
33. Gerberding JL, Falk H, Arias I, et al. In a moment's notice: surge capacity for terrorist bombings challenges and proposed solutions. In: Services USDoHaH, editor. 2007. p. 60. http://emergency.cdc.gov/masscasualties/pdf/surgecapacity.pdf.
34. Kelen GD, McCarthy ML. The science of surge. Acad Emerg Med. 2006;13(11):1089–94.
35. Abramovich MN, Hershey JC, Callies B, Adalja AA, Tosh PK, Toner ES. Hospital influenza pandemic stockpiling needs: a computer simulation. Am J Infect Control. 2017;45(3):272–7.
36. Posner Z, Admi H, Menashe N. Ten-fold expansion of a burn unit in mass casualty: how to recruit the nursing staff. Disaster Manag Response. 2003;1(4):100–4.
37. Lennarson P, Boedeker BH, Kuper GM, et al. Utilization of a civilian academic center as a force multiplier in support of NATO special operations medicine—a pilot demonstration. Stud Health Technol Inform. 2012;173:260–2.
38. Bryan J, Miyamoto D, Holman V. Medical civil-military operations: the deployed medical brigade's role in counterinsurgency operations. US Army Med Dep J. 2008;25–28.
39. Simmons S, Alverson D, Poropatich R, D'Iorio J, DeVany M, Doarn CR. Applying telehealth in natural and anthropogenic disasters. Telemed J E Health. 2008;14(9):968–71.
40. Franco C, Toner E, Waldhorn R, Inglesby TV, O'Toole T. The national disaster medical system: past, present, and suggestions for the future. Biosecur Bioterror. 2007;5(4):319–25.
41. Kearns RD, Conlon KM, Valenta AL, Lord GC, Cairns CB, Holmes JH, Johnson DD, Matherly AF, Sawyer D, Skarote MB, Siler SM, Helminiak RC, Cairns BA. Disaster planning: the basics of creating a burn mass casualty disaster plan for a burn center. J Burn Care Res. 2014;35(1):e1–e13. https://doi.org/10.1097/BCR.0b013e31829afe25. PubMed PMID: 23877135.
42. Franc JM, Ingrassia PL, Verde M, Colombo D, Della Corte F. A simple graphical method for quantification of disaster management surge capacity using computer simulation and process-control tools. Prehosp Disaster Med. 2015;30(1):9–15.
43. Toerper MF, Kelen GD, Sauer LM, Bayram JD, Catlett C, Levin S. Hospital surge capacity: a web-based simulation tool for emergency planners. Disaster Med Public Health Prep. 2018;12(4):513–22.
44. Nilsson H, Jonson CO, Vikstrom T, et al. Simulation-assisted burn disaster planning. Burns. 2013;39(6):1122–30.
45. Abir M, Davis MM, Sankar P, Wong AC, Wang SC. Design of a model to predict surge capacity bottlenecks for burn mass casualties at a large academic medical center. Prehosp Disaster Med. 2013;28(1):23–32.
46. Albores P, Shaw D. Government preparedness: using simulation to prepare for a terrorist attack. Comput Oper Res. 2008;35(6):1924–43.
47. Dallas CE, Bell WC. Prediction modeling to determine the adequacy of medical response to urban nuclear attack. Disaster Med Public Health Prep. 2007;1(2):80–9.
48. Franc-Law JM, Bullard M, Della Corte F. Simulation of a hospital disaster plan: a virtual, live exercise. Prehosp Disaster Med. 2008;23(4):346–53.
49. Hirshberg A, Scott BG, Granchi T, Wall MJ, Mattox KL, Stein M. How does casualty load affect trauma care in urban bombing incidents? A quantitative analysis. J Trauma. 2005;58(4):686–95.
50. Smith SW, Portelli I, Narzisi G, et al. A novel approach to multihazard modeling and simulation. Disaster Med Public Health Prep. 2009;3(2):75–87.
51. Steward D, Wan TT. The role of simulation and modeling in disaster management. J Med Syst. 2007;31(2):125–30.

52. Kearns R, Zoller J, Hubble M, Alson R, Cairns B, Holmes J IV. Using Monte Carlo simulation for modeling surge capacity in the ABA southern region. J Burn Care Res. 2012;33(2):1.
53. Kearns RD. Burn surge capacity in the south what is the capacity of burn centers within the american burn association southern region to absorb significant numbers of burn injured patients during a medical disaster? Medical University of South Carolina: ProQuest Dissertations and Theses; 2011.
54. Agency FEMA. Homeland security exercise and evaluation program. 2013. http://www.fema.gov/media-library-data/20130726-1914-25045-8890/hseep_apr13_.pdf. Accessed 6 July 2016.

Common Wounding Mechanisms and Injury Patterns

3

Miklosh Bala and Jeffry Kashuk

3.1 Introduction

Terrorist attacks, as a mechanism of injury, continue to be a worldwide challenge to trauma centers, resulting in tremendous and varied injury patterns often in large numbers of victims. While terrorists may use many different approaches to inflict injury, explosive devices, often homemade, have continued to be the prime weaponry for terror-related events. These attacks create mass-casualty emergencies and trigger unique pattern of injuries which require a detailed understanding by the treatment team in order to provide optimal care. Other commonly used injury mechanisms include gunshots and knives. Finally, blunt trauma in terror-related MCI may be caused by stoning and intentional road accidents (car ramming).

Historically, terrorist attacks worldwide have been characterized by continued changes by terrorists in their evil attempts to inflict injury. For example, the most recent experiences with terror events in Israel, since September 2000, have mainly involved suicide bomber explosions (54% of the hospitalized victims) and gunshots (36% of the hospitalized victims) [1, 2].

Interestingly, in the time frame of 2000–2004, suicide bombers comprised less than 1% of attacks but claimed 47% of the fatalities, while in the Jerusalem region, 60% of hospitalized patients at Hadassah University Hospital sustained gunshot wounds as opposed to bomb explosion mechanisms [3].

Because blast injury is clearly the most lethal mechanism in terrorist attacks, it is incumbent on the practitioner treating such injuries to acquire essential knowledge of the injury patterns noted in an MCI. Such knowledge is integrally tied to

M. Bala (✉)
Trauma and Acute Care Surgery Unit, Hadassah—Hebrew University Medical Center, Jerusalem, Israel
e-mail: rbalam@hadassah.org.il

J. Kashuk
Assia Medical Group, Tel Aviv University-Sackler School of Medicine, Tel Aviv, Israel

Y. Kluger et al. (eds.), *WSES Handbook of Mass Casualties Incidents Management*, Hot Topics in Acute Care Surgery and Trauma,
https://doi.org/10.1007/978-3-319-92345-1_3

treatment plans, and therefore, is an essential aspect of trauma care in terrorist scenarios. Accordingly, the initial focus of this chapter will be to review injury mechanisms in bomb explosions. Other relevant injury mechanisms will be discussed too.

3.2 Type of Wounding Mechanism

3.2.1 Explosions

Bodily injuries induced by explosive blasts have been characterized as primary, secondary, tertiary, and quaternary injuries. When an explosive device detonates, a relatively small volume of explosive is rapidly transformed into a large volume of gas. A high-pressure blast wave quickly spreads out at the speed of sound, and its interaction with the body causes primary blast injuries (mainly involving air-filled and hollow organs such as the lung, ear, and bowel). In air, this shock wave dissolves rapidly, in relation to the cube of the distance from the blast. When the shock wave passes through the body, the tissue disruption occurs most significantly at air–liquid interfaces. The degree of tissue injury is directly related to the magnitude and the duration of the peak overpressure of the blast shock wave (Fig. 3.1).

The peak and duration of overpressure represent the amount of energy transferred to surrounding medium. Following this, a longer phase of negative pressure is encountered, leading to a tremendous wave of air known as "blast wave."

The blast wave creates a wounding mechanism due to its ability to push solid materials along with the wave. These may be intentionally placed within the bomb by terrorists, or can be recruited from the surrounding environment (concrete, stones, glass). Impaction of such materials in the human body may lead to injuries which simulate penetrating injury mechanisms (secondary injury). Alternatively, the force of the shock wave may propel a person into a solid object, creating an injury pattern similar to blunt trauma. Lastly, the inhalation of smoke and hot gases

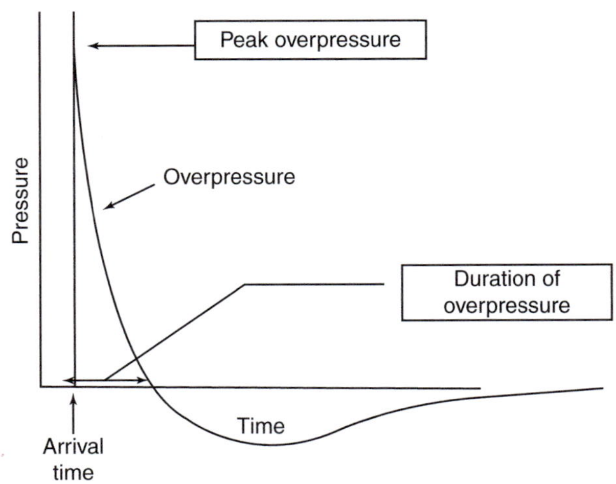

Fig. 3.1 Pressure–time graph of blast wave

Table 3.1 Mechanisms of blast injury

Category	Characteristics	Body part affected	Types of injuries
Primary	Results from the impact of an over-pressurization wave with body surfaces	Gas filled structures are most susceptible – Lungs, GI tract, and middle ear	– Blast lung (pulmonary barotrauma) – TM rupture and middle ear damage – Abdominal hemorrhage and perforation – Globe (eye) rupture – Concussion (TBI without physical signs of head injury)
Secondary	Results from flying debris and bomb fragments	Any body part may be affected	– Penetrating ballistic (fragmentation)
Tertiary	Results from individuals being thrown by the blast wind	Any body part may be affected	– Fracture and traumatic amputation – Closed and open brain injury
Quaternary	All explosion-related injuries, diseases not due to primary, secondary, or tertiary mechanisms	Any body part may be affected	– Burns – Crush injuries – Asthma, COPD, or other breathing problems from dust, smoke, or toxic fumes – Angina – Hypertension

causes injuries and exposure to heat, flames, and dust and have been termed quaternary injury. This phenomenon when different classes of injury occur simultaneously in the same patient was termed multidimensional injury pattern [4] (Table 3.1).

The existing literature recognizes the influence of the type of environment where an explosion occurs on the outcomes of the injured, mostly differentiating between closed and open spaces [5–9]. Due to the physics of explosions, those occurring within enclosed settings will have a greater impact because of the amplification of the blast through reflection from the surrounding environment. In particular, bus explosions have a high lethality as they represent a "classic" closed space, often with many potential victims in close proximity [5, 10, 11].

Peleg and others have reported that the profiles of the five explosion types to be significantly different from each other both in terms of sustained injuries, their treatment, and the consequent clinical outcomes [12]. The enclosed space was separated to explosion inside the building or bus (inside the bus or adjacent to it) or open space explosion: close to building (semi-open space) or pure open space. Regarding injury parameters, the new taxonomy was found to be more precise than that of the traditional three category classification to "open," "closed," and "semi-closed" settings.

3.2.2 Flying Missiles Wounds (Secondary Blast Injuries)

In addition to the pure blast effect, new injury mechanisms introduced by terrorism included penetrating injuries by different size metal pieces, such as nails, screws, pellets, and bolts, that are inserted into the bomb and are propelled with extreme force following explosion. Many such metal pieces, penetrating an individual simultaneously, result in extremely devastating and challenging injuries. The ability to identify penetrations that often leave only minor entry wounds, concealed by hair or clothes, is limited. These obscured wounds might seem minor, but are often associated with severe internal damage (Fig. 3.2).

Diagnostic imaging is necessary to map the routes and the extent of injury. Use of imaging modalities, such as CT scans and focused abdominal ultrasonography, in trauma was considerably greater in blast injuries, reflecting a complex but less defined and localized type of injury [13]. Liberal use of imaging techniques was justified by the need to search for internal injuries that are not identified on physical examination. Experience has taught us that the strength of impact and the tract taken by secondary missiles within the patient's body are unpredictable [14]. Unlike an injury caused by gunshot, where entrance and exit wounds tend to be visible. For this reason, use of CT scans for accurate and rapid diagnosis of penetrating injuries has been added to the protocol for dealing with blast injuries in our institution [15].

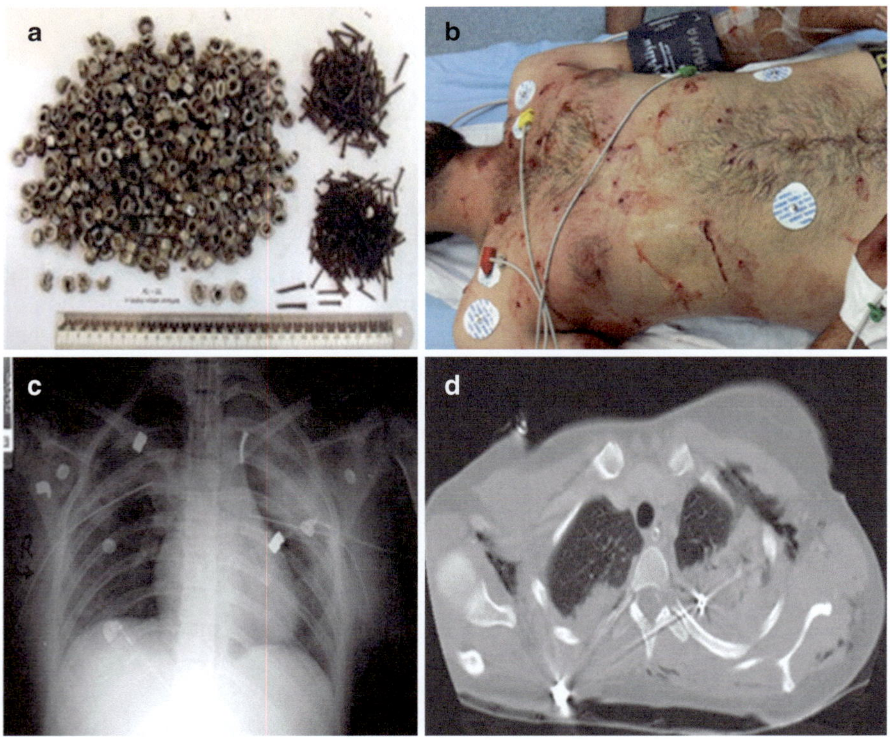

Fig. 3.2 Flying missiles from bombs (**a**) and multiple skin abrasions caused by small flying objects or debris (**b**). The same patient's chest X-ray (**c**) and CT scan show multiple foreign bodies in chest wall and lung (**d**)

Furthermore, debridement of each and every entry wound is time-consuming and may not always be justified, especially when taking into account the limited resources at the time of a large influx of patients.

3.2.3 Gunshot Wounds

In the recent experience in Israel, gunshot wounds often occur from snipers shooting at pedestrians or drivers. As such, these shootings are well aimed at vital organs such as the head and the chest and are often fatal. The patients who arrive alive at the hospital after a shooting incident usually have longer transportation time in comparison to victims of explosion attacks [3]. Blast injuries, in contrast with gunshot events, are typically associated with mass casualty incidents that usually takes place in an urban setting. Also patients with gunshot wounds are often transferred directly to the operating room for immediate operation, without earlier use of imaging. Gunshot wounds are usually isolated cases.

Accordingly, the mortality for GSW in the terrorist setting has been higher than in conventional scenarios. Of note, such injuries were primarily in young (60% aged 19–30 years) and male (90%) victims. This is explained by the fact that members of the main group injured by this mechanism were soldiers (34.4%), drivers, or tourists in isolated regions [13].

3.3 Injury Patterns Following Explosions

The range of injuries sustained by victims of suicide bombing attacks (SBAs) is more complex and more severe compared with victims of other forms of trauma [16]. Victims will typically suffer from blast lung injury (BLI), penetrating missiles, blunt trauma, and burns. Severe injuries (ISS > 16) were reported in 28.7% of victims of terrorist explosions compared with 10% of victims of other forms of trauma [4].

3.3.1 Head Injuries

The brain is clearly vulnerable to all blast injury (caused by primary blast, flying debris, and fragments) and tertiary blast injury (caused by being thrown by blast wind). Although prior reports questioned whether the brain may be susceptible to primary blast injury (caused by the overpressure wave), animal models suggest this indeed to be the case [17]. Shear and stress waves from the overpressure explosion wave may lead to traumatic brain injury (e.g., concussion, hemorrhage, edema, and diffuse axonal injury) [18]. The primary blast mechanism can also result in cerebral infarction due to blast lung injury and consequent formation of gas emboli [19]. Subarachnoid and subdural hemorrhages are the most common findings in fatalities [20, 21]. In contrast, the majority of injuries in survivors have been due to penetrating missiles [22]. Experience from Israel has shown that the head is the most

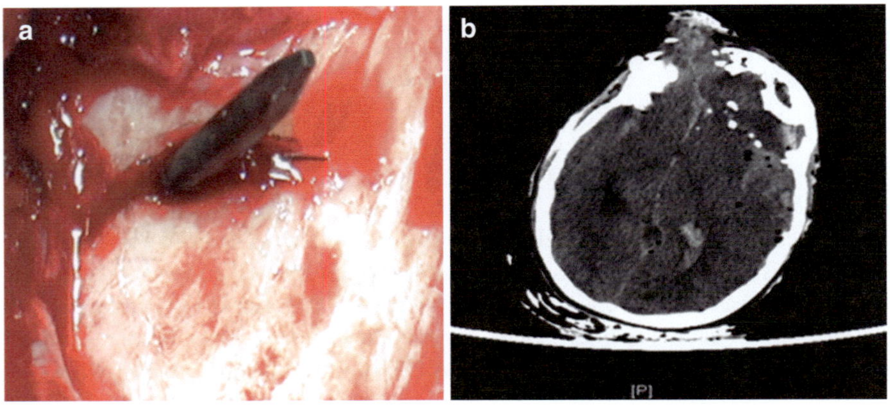

Fig. 3.3 Penetrating skull injuries following bombing attack. Nail in the skull (**a**). CT scan of head with penetrating injury caused by flying missile following blast injury (**b**)

frequent site of penetrating wounds and that 29–54.5% of victims suffer from penetrating injury to the head [1, 23] (Fig. 3.3).

As previously stated, blast waves can cause concussion or mild traumatic brain injury. Studies have shown that primary blast injury to the brain results in damaged glial cells and a pronounced vagal state leading to sustained hypotension and bradycardia [24].

Higher levels of blast overpressure can cause skull fractures. Indeed, the presence of skull fractures in the face of blast injury was found to be a clue to the presence of BLI [25].

3.3.2 Lung and Chest Injuries

BLI is a major cause of immediate death and morbidity. It can occur without external chest wall injury, caused by the very high-pressure primary blast wave pushing the chest wall towards the spine, causing transient high intrathoracic pressure [26]. Among the casualties recorded in Israel as suffering from an injury from bomb blasts, 21% had a lung injury—17.5% severe (AIS 3 or above) and 3.7% of minor severity. In the Jerusalem terrorist attacks, one medical center reported that more than half (52%) of the patients in the intensive care unit (ICU) had lung injuries [27]. Of the ICU patients with blast lung, 21% had combined chest and head injuries and 11% had combined chest and abdominal injuries [28]. External injury to four or more body regions was found to be a predictor of blast lung and intra-abdominal injuries [29].

BLI is a very complex injury to manage and requires advanced critical care techniques to balance between low-pressure ventilation and satisfactory oxygenation (Fig. 3.4).

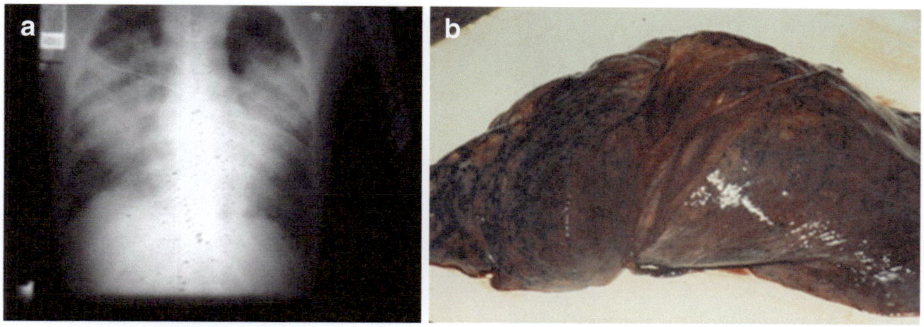

Fig. 3.4 Typical X-ray (**a**) of severe blast lung injury showing typical bilateral patchy lung infiltrates ("butterfly" pattern). Macroscopic picture of blast lung from patient injures inside the bus (**b**). Severe edema and parenchymal hemorrhage are seen. Reprinted with permission from Almogy G, Rivkind AI. Terror in the 21st century: milestones and prospects--part I. Curr Probl Surg. 2007;44:496–554. Copyright Elsevier 2018

3.3.3 Auditory Injury

The ear is the organ most sensitive to blast injury. Auditory injury has been reported in 35–41% of survivors of bombing attacks [30]. Blast overpressure tears sensory cells from the basilar membrane, which eventually heals with scar leading to prolonged disability from hearing loss [31]. The explosion setting will determine the frequency of auditory injury and ranges from 8% in open spaces to 50% in confined spaces [4].

Controversy exists regarding the significance of tympanic membrane (TM) rupture as a predictor of occult BLI. In a recent review, the authors advocated the value of routine otoscopy in triaging victims of terror bombing attacks to identify those suspected with severe blast lung injury [32]. Others have not found such a significant role for such screening. Leibovici and colleagues reported on 647 victims of 11 terrorist bombing attacks [33]. Of the 49 victims who suffered from BLI, 18 (36.7%) had no TM rupture at all. Similar experience from Hadassah Trauma Unit showed that of the 154 victims who were admitted for more than 24 h, 34 (22.1%) had TM rupture but it was not necessarily associated with BLI. Of note, however, TM rupture appears to be associated with BLI in confined spaces such as buses [34].

3.3.4 Abdominal Injuries

Abdominal injury associated with terrorist explosions has been shown to occur in 10% of victims admitted to a tertiary care hospital [35]. The most common mechanisms were penetrating wounds caused by shrapnel and flying debris (96%). Primary hollow viscous injuries include hemorrhage, petechia, and circumferential rings of hemorrhage. Transmural lesions can lead to bowel perforation, hemoperitoneum, peritonitis, and sepsis. Perforations may develop up to 24–48 h later; however,

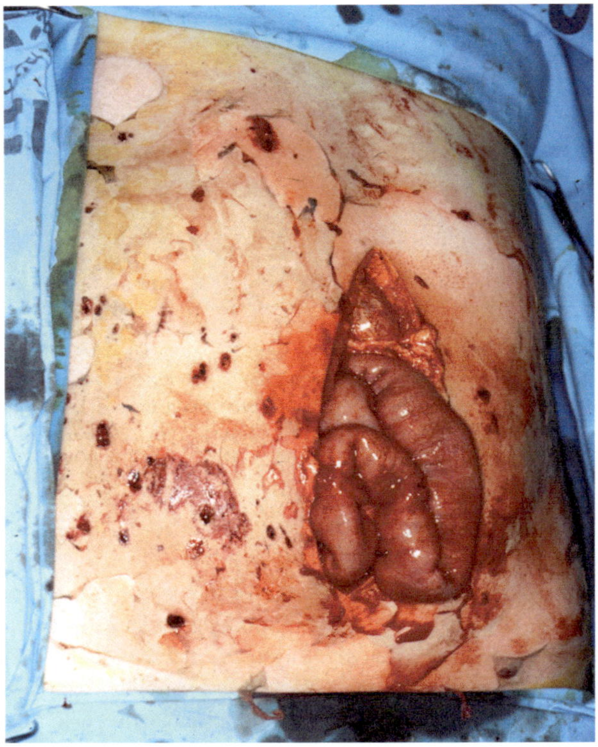

Fig. 3.5 Multiple bowel injuries caused by secondary blast mechanism

delays of up to 14 days have been reported [36]. Abdominal injury caused by the blast wave is uncommon and only a few cases had been reported [11, 37].

Nearly, a third of the patients in the ICU due to bomb explosions suffered an abdominal injury [27]. Only a small portion of these were solely secondary to blast or blunt injuries (4%), while 21% were a combination of blunt and penetrating injuries.

Most patients with significant abdominal trauma underwent explorative laparotomy. Only a minority were placed under observation. Bowel injury was found in 71.4% of blast victims, more often than in GSW and blunt trauma [38] (Fig. 3.5).

3.3.5 Orthopedic Injuries

Skeletal injuries inflicted by terrorism are described by Weil et al., who described several modes of severe penetrating injuries causing high-grade open fractures [39].

Gunshot wounds and multiple penetrating injuries following blast trauma caused by terrorism produce complex penetrating long bone injuries, often associated with multiple trauma. In a study of 85 orthopedic patients from 33 terrorist attacks in Jerusalem, 113 long bone fractures caused by penetrating gunshot and shrapnel injuries were recorded. There were 36 femoral fractures, 50 tibial fractures, 5 humeral fractures, and 24 forearm fractures. Thirty-six percent of the patients had multiple fractures, while 43% suffered from significant associated injuries, mainly vascular damage and/or nerve injury to the fractured extremity [27].

Traumatic amputations are the consequence of blast overpressures and high velocity shock waves and are often associated with a poor prognosis. Of the 74 victims with traumatic amputations reported by Almogy and colleagues, 63 (85.1%) died at the scene [25].

3.3.6 Soft Tissue Injuries

In many terrorist bombings, there is an overwhelming predominance of relatively minor injuries that are not life threatening [40, 41]. The area of the victim's body facing the explosion presents "peppering" of the skin consisting of subcutaneous hemorrhages, abrasions, and superficial and deep lacerations, a characteristic triad in explosion victims [42] (Fig. 3.6). These are usually caused by secondary and tertiary blast effects and are typically soft tissue and skeletal injuries that may tend to be contaminated and require multiple debridement procedures.

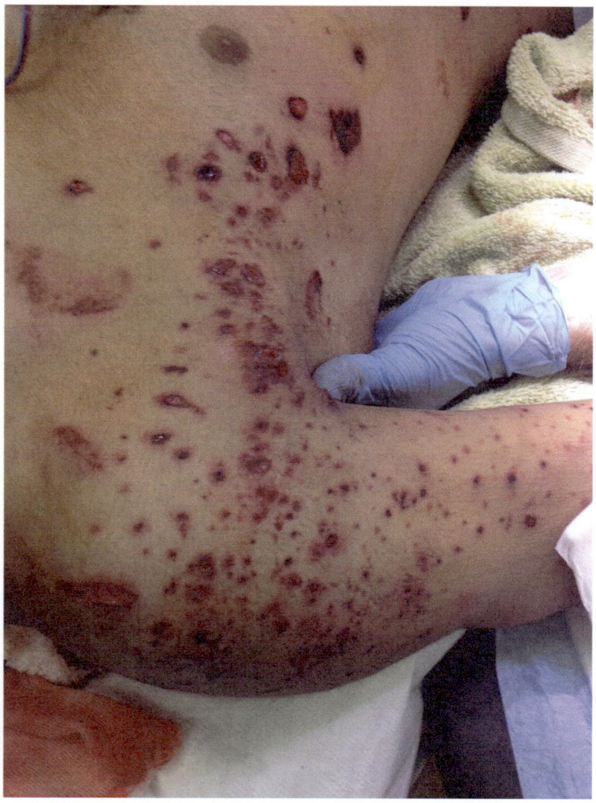

Fig. 3.6 Skin laceration in blast trauma victim. "Peppering" of the skin consisting of subcutaneous hemorrhages, abrasions, and superficial and deep lacerations

After the terrorist attacks in Madrid in 2004, soft tissue, musculoskeletal, and ear blast injuries predominated in up to 80% of the cases, but were mostly noncritical in severity and contributed little to mortality [43]. The main problem with these minor injuries is that the multiple-contaminated wounds contain various debris and fragments. The wound debridement in these patients is necessary to prevent subsequent infection [44]. In Spain, such injuries accounted for more than a third of all operations performed in the first 24 h. Standard procedure in Israel is to avoid the hunt for each piece of shrapnel. Imbedded metal fragments are removed if they are found at the time of exploration, or if their close proximity to a vital organ may carry potential danger or may potentially lead to irreversible damage [45].

3.3.7 Burns

Thermal injuries from explosions of conventional weapons are classified as quaternary blast injuries. The rapidly expanding fireball from the explosion may cause flash burns over exposed body parts (e.g., hands, neck, and head). Confined space explosions can enhance thermal effects and increase the risk of inhalation injury (Fig. 3.7).

Effectively managing thermal injuries associated with primary blast injury, particularly blast lung injury, may be challenging due to conflicting fluid requirements.

Terror-attack injuries with accompanying burns have a more complex presentation, are of higher severity, and are associated with increased length of hospital stay and a higher ICU admissions rate, compared with terror-attack injuries without burns and non-terror-attack related burns. Interestingly, mortality rates in terror-attack injuries are not affected by burns. Most bomb-related burns cover <20% of the total body surface area, but occur in combination with other blast injuries. Of note, however, burns over 30% in combination with other blast injuries almost never survive [25]. On the other hand, inhalation injury is relatively common (18%) among those who survive explosions in confined spaces [1].

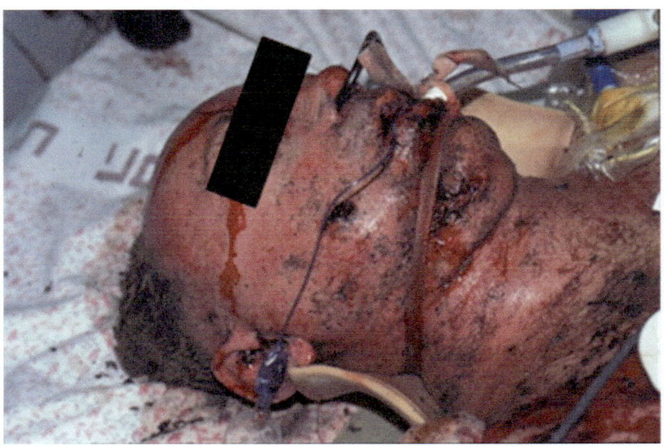

Fig. 3.7 A 22-year-old serviceman following blast injury with severe burn injury to the face and inhalation

Burn-terror patients have a significantly higher injury severity score compared with no-burn/terror group, but a mortality rate of 6.4% was similar in both groups [46].

3.4 Perpetrator Bone Fragment Injuries

Braverman et al. report on another unusual but problematic aspect of suicide bombings: the penetration of bone fragments from the human suicide bomber [47]. In this report, the perpetrator had hepatitis B and the bone fragments were positive for hepatitis B surface antigen HbsAG, resulting in the need to administer active immunization against hepatitis B for all the patients injured in the attack. Hospital preparedness protocol was changed accordingly for further MCIs. Current protocol is that in each case of suicide bombing, all victims are vaccinated for hepatitis B. Of note, however, none had active viral infection.

3.5 Mechanism of Injury in Recent MCI's

A recent new wave of terror in Middle East and later in Europe brings other challenging MCI's scenarios as opposed to wounds caused by suicide bombers.

3.5.1 Stabbing

Stabbing has long been an instrument of traumatic assault, as knifes are easily obtainable and effective killing instruments.

The mortality rate associated with stabbing is reported to be relatively low (<5%) in comparison to high energy weapons [48]. The current reality, however, requires that trauma units be prepared for the unique characteristics of terrorist stabbings. The most prominent increase in knife terror in the recent years was the so called "Knife Intifada" in Israel, when multiple stabbing attacks were perpetrated against Israeli serviceman and civilians as a primary target from October 2015 to March 2016 [49]. Producing multiple victims, these attacks once again reminded the trauma physicians in Israel that their previous experience of dealing with non-terror stabbings could differ extensively from the injuries of knife terror patients [50].

The likely explanation for this disparity is the non-personal nature of terror attacks—the attacker frequently runs trying to stab as many people as possible, without any previous acquaintance with the victims. Head, neck, and upper torso injuries became the hallmark of these events. Prehospital medical teams had to deal with non-compressible life-threatening injuries and the quick evacuation to the designated trauma centers became a key point in management of these injuries.

3.5.2 Intentional Vehicular Assaults

Injury caused by a motor vehicle driven intentionally into a pedestrian crowd has recently become another method of terrorism. This method of attack was first seen in Israel in 1987 when a car was intentionally driven into a group of soldiers inflicting severe injuries. Over the past decades, there have been many random attacks, and unfortunately, the world has experienced these in other regions as well (Nice, Berlin, London, and others). During the 3-month time frame, from September 2015, 43 such attacks were recorded in Jerusalem only. We have adopted the term "intentional vehicular assault" (IVA) to describe this specific type of terror attack.

A new type of terrorist attack, the lone terrorist attacker, has become more frequent recently and includes IVA and stabbing attacks. This "lone wolf" phenomenon is characterized by radicals who embark on individual terrorist missions with little or no logistical support [51].

To date, these attacks have occurred mostly in the Middle East and Europe. In Israel, most attacks have centered on the greater Jerusalem area, mainly due to ease of access and insufficiency in security settings. The majority involved civilian cars although some used heavy construction equipment, making the attacks more lethal. Of note, two recent attacks involved a combination of a vehicle strike, followed by stabbing.

Of significance, we have noted that the pattern and severity of injury following IVA is significantly different from non-terror pedestrian injury [52] with a significantly higher ISS due to more severe head injuries leading to higher mortality.

On the basis of video clips and witness reports, deliberate vehicular towards an upright pedestrian may lead to high energy trauma to the lower extremities as well as severe head trauma. Indeed, we noted this injury pattern in the IVA group [52].

The median number of casualties who were admitted to the ED following an IVA was relatively small (range of 1–10 victims per attack) when compared with the number of casualties following other types of terror acts such as suicide bombing attacks. On the other hand, IVA events resulted in multiple casualties have certainly occurred in Israel and worldwide. In one event, 70 casualties occurred when a bulldozer rammed into a crowd on a Jerusalem main street (Fig. 3.8), and there were more than 200 casualties following the Nice (France) attack (July 14, 2016) which involved a truck.

3.5.3 Active Shooter Incidents

On June 12, 2016, a gunman entered a nightclub in Orlando with military-grade weapons, leaving 49 dead and 53 wounded.

The incidence and severity of civilian public mass shootings continues to shock the world. Initiatives predicated on lessons learned from military experience have placed strong emphasis on hemorrhage control, especially via use of tourniquets, as a potential means to improve survival.

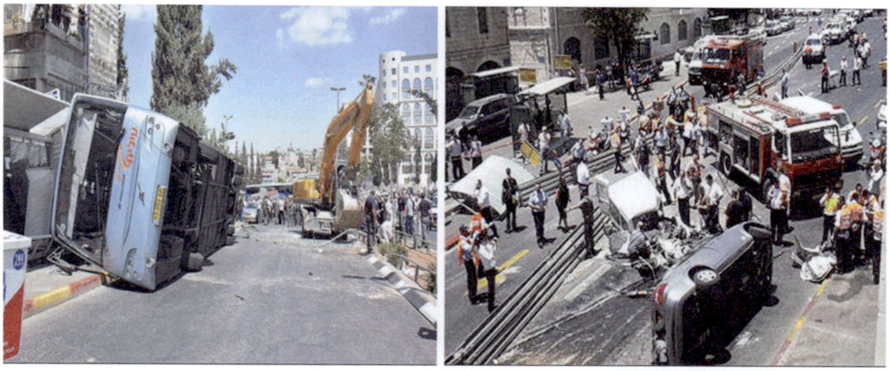

Fig. 3.8 The scene of IVA with serious damage to public area by industrial vehicle used as a "weapon." The perpetrator rammed his bulldozer into cars and a bus on King David Street in Jerusalem on July 22, 2008. He wounded 24 people

It should be emphasized, however, that the difference in the anatomic regions of wounds between combat and civilian public mass shootings is quite significant. The percentage of extremity injuries in combat has been reported to be between 52 and 64% [53]. In contrast, an analysis of 12 shooting events in US showed that only 28 of 139 total civilians (20%) had extremity wounds of any kind. Instead, civilians have a much higher percentage of head and torso injuries (72% versus 48% in combat) [54]. The likely reason for this is that the civilians are not wearing ballistic protection for their head and/or torso leading to a higher incidence of injury to these anatomic regions. Civilian public mass shootings most often occur at a much closer range and most often indoors [55]. Also, the closer distance in civilian settings greatly improves the accuracy and ability for the shooter to hit center mass, thus creating a higher incidence of head and torso injuries.

Civilian public mass shootings overall are more lethal events with a significantly higher case fatality rate than combat. The case fatality rate (CFR) for 12 events summarized by Smith et al. [54], defined as the percentage of fatalities among all wounded, was 44.6% [56]. Overall, from 2000 to 2013, the CFR for active shooting events as reported by the FBI was 46.5% [57]. In contrast, during Operation Iraqi Freedom, the CFR has been reported in certain military groups to be 9–10% [58]. Trauma management training models based upon the prior military experience is a valuable exercise to aid medical knowledge in civilian response to high threat events.

Conclusions

In this chapter, we have outlined the common mechanisms of injuries during mass casualty incidents. As terrorists continue to attempt new and different wounding mechanisms, trauma systems must be prepared for the influx of casualties. Current experience suggest that prior experience with conventional gunshot wounds, stabbing attacks, and motor vehicle collisions may underestimate the severity of injury when compared to terror attacks. The range of injuries sustained by victims of suicide bombing attacks is more complex and more severe compared with victims of other forms of trauma. It is crucial to recognize that victims of suicide bombing attacks are potentially injured by four different mechanisms. Victims will typically suffer from blast lung injury, penetrating missiles, blunt trauma, and burns. The majority of victims of penetrating trauma (firearms) sustain injuries to isolated parts of the body such as the head, chest, abdomen, or limbs. Blunt trauma is more commonly a multisite injury, the severity of which depends on the mechanism of injury. The multidimensional injury patient will often require the careful coordination of multiple surgical teams. But in such a scenario, the trauma surgeon must remain the "captain of the ship," prioritizing care and determining appropriate application of damage control principles.

The world terror epidemic is a continuous and pressing challenge to our trauma systems, and shared knowledge and experience as well as an understanding of wounding mechanisms is essential for improved survival in this group.

References

1. Peleg K, Aharonson-Daniel L, Stein M, Shapira SC. Patterns of injury in hospitalized terrorist victims. Am J Emerg Med. 2003;21:258–62.
2. Israel Defense Forces Web site. http://www.idf.il/. Accessed 30 Jan 2018.
3. Sheffy N, Mintz Y, Rivkind A, Shapira SC. Terror-related injuries: a comparison of gunshot wounds versus secondary-fragments—induced injuries from explosives. J Am Coll Surg. 2006;203:297–303.
4. Kluger Y, Peleg K, Daniel-Aharonson L, Mayo A, Israeli Trauma Group. The special injury pattern in terrorist bombings. J Am Coll Surg. 2004;199:875–9.
5. Champion HR, Holcomb JB, Young LA. Injuries from explosions: physics, bio-physics, pathology, and required research focus. J Trauma. 2009;66:1468–77.
6. Kosashvili Y, Loebenberg MI, Lin G, et al. Medical consequences of suicide bombing mass casualty incidents: the impact of explosion setting on injury patterns. Injury. 2009;40:698–702.
7. Leibovici D, Gofrit ON, Stein M, et al. Blast injuries: bus versus open-air bombings—a comparative study of injuries in survivors of open-air versus confined-space explosions. J Trauma. 1996;41:1030–5.
8. Arnold JL, Halpern P, Tsai M-C, et al. Mass casualty terrorist bombings: a comparison of outcomes by bombing type. Ann Emerg Med. 2004;43:263–73.
9. Wolf SJ, Bebarta VS, Bonnett CJ, et al. Blast injuries. Lancet. 2009;374:405–15.
10. Golan R, Soffer D, Givon A, et al. The ins and outs of terrorist bus explosions: injury profiles of on-board explosions versus explosions occurring adjacent to a bus. Injury. 2014;45:39–43.
11. Katz E, Ofek B, Adler J, et al. Primary blast injury after a bomb explosion in a civilian bus. Ann Surg. 1989;209:484–8.
12. Rozenfeld M, Givon A, Shenhar G, Renert L, Peleg K. A new paradigm of injuries from terrorist explosions as a function of explosion setting type. Ann Surg. 2016;263:1228–34.
13. Almogy G, Bala M, Rivkind A. The approach to suicide bombing attacks: changing concepts. Eur J Trauma Emerg Surg. 2007;33:641–7.
14. Kashuk JL, Halperin P, Caspi G, Colwell C, Moore EE. Bomb explosions in acts of terrorism: evil creativity challenges our trauma systems. J Am Coll Surg. 2009;209:134–40.
15. Sosna J, Sella T, Shaham D, Shapira SC, Rivkind A, Bloom AI, Libson E. Facing the new threats of terrorism: radiologists' perspectives based on experience in Israel. Radiology. 2005;237:28–36.

16. Peleg K, Savitsky B, Israeli Trauma Group. Terrorism-related injuries versus road traffic accident-related trauma: 5 years of experience in Israel. Disaster Med Public Health Prep. 2009;3:196–200.
17. Cernak I, Merkle AC, Koliatsos VE, Bilik JM, Luong QT, Mahota TM, Xu L, Slack N, Windle D, Ahmed FA. The pathobiology of blast injuries and blast-induced neurotrauma as identified using a new experimental model of injury in mice. Neurobiol Dis. 2011;41:538–51.
18. Goldstein LE, Fisher AM, Tagge CA, Zhang XL, Velisek L, Sullivan JA, et al. Chronic traumatic encephalopathy in blast-exposed military veterans and a blast neurotrauma mouse model. Sci Transl Med. 2012;4:134ra60.
19. Lipschutz JH, Pascuzzi RM, Bognanno J, Putty T. Bilateral anterior cerebral artery infarction resulting from explosion-type injury to the head and neck. Stroke. 1991;22:813–5.
20. Cernak I. The importance of systemic response in the pathobiology of blast-induced neurotrauma. Front Neurol. 2010;1:1–9.
21. Hill JF. Blast injury with particular reference to recent terrorist bombing incidents. Ann R Coll Surg Engl. 1979;61:4–11.
22. Rosenthal G, Roemi L, Shoshan Y, Segal R, Umansky F. Penetrating head injuries from terrorist bomb blasts: the Jerusalem experience. Presented as an abstract at the Congress of Neurological Surgeons. San Francisco, CA, October 2004.
23. Aharonson-Daniel L, Klein Y, Peleg K. Suicide bombers form a new injury profile. Ann Surg. 2006;244:1018–23.
24. Cernak I, Wang Z, Jiang J, et al. Ultrastructural and functional characteristics of blast injury-induced neurotrauma. J Trauma. 2001;50:695–706.
25. Almogy G, Luria T, Richter E, Pizov R, Bdolah-Abram T, Mintz Y, et al. Can external signs of trauma guide management? Lessons learned from suicide bombing attacks in Israel. Arch Surg. 2004;140:390–3.
26. Hare SS, Goddard I, Ward P, Naraghi A, Dick EA. The radiological management of bomb blast injury. Clin Radiol. 2007;62:1–9.
27. Aschkenasy-Steuer G, Shamir M, Rivkind A, Mosheiff R, Shushan Y, Rosenthal G, Mintz Y, Weissman C, Sprung CL, Weiss YG. Clinical review: the Israeli experience: conventional terrorism and critical care. Crit Care. 2005;9:490–9.
28. Avidan V, Hersch M, Spira RM, Einav S, Goldberg S, Schecter W. Civilian hospital response to a mass casualty event: the role of the intensive care unit. J Trauma. 2007;62:1234–9.
29. Almogy G, Belzberg H, Mintz Y, et al. Suicide bombing attacks: update and modifications to the protocol. Ann Surg. 2004;239:295–303.
30. Wightman J, Gladish S. Explosions and blast injuries. Ann Emerg Med. 2001;37:664–78.
31. Patterson J, Hamernik R. Blast overpressure induced structural and functional changes the auditory system. Toxicology. 1997;121:29–40.
32. DePalma RG, Burris DG, Champion HR, Hodgson MJ. Current concepts: blast injuries. N Engl J Med. 2005;352:1335–42.
33. Leibovici D, Gofrit ON, Shapira SC. Eardrum perforation in explosion survivors: is it a marker of pulmonary blast injury? Ann Emerg Med. 1999;34:168–72.
34. Hirshberg B, Oppenheim-Eden A, Pizov R, et al. Recovery from blast lung injury. One year follow-up. Chest. 1999;116:1683–8.
35. Almogy G, Mintz Y, Zamir G, et al. Suicide bombing attacks: can external signs predict internal injuries? Ann Surg. 2006;243:541–6.
36. Singer P, Cohen J, Stein M. Conventional terrorism and critical care. Crit Care Med. 2005;33(1 Suppl):S61–5.
37. Paran H, Neufeld D, Shwartz I, et al. Perforation of the terminal ileum induced by blast injury: delayed diagnosis or delayed perforation. J Trauma. 1996;40:472–5.
38. Bala M, Rivkind AI, Zamir G, Hadar T, Gertsenshtein I, Mintz Y, Pikarsky AJ, Amar D, Shussman N, Abu Gazala M, Almogy G. Abdominal trauma after terrorist bombing attacks exhibits a unique pattern of injury. Ann Surg. 2008;248:303–9.
39. Weil YA, Petrov K, Liebergal M, Mintz Y, Mosheiff R. Long bone fractures caused by penetrating injuries in terrorists attacks. J Trauma. 2007;62:909–12.

40. Feliciano DV, Anderson GV, Rozycki GS, et al. Management of casualties from the bombing at the Centennial Olympics. Am J Surg. 1998;176:538–43.
41. Frykberg ER. Medical management of disasters and mass casualties from terrorist bombings: how can we cope? J Trauma. 2002;53:201–12.
42. Saukko P, Knight B. Gunshot and explosion deaths in: Knight's forensic pathology. 3rd ed. London: Arnold; 2004. p. 245–80.
43. de Ceballos JP, Turegano-Fuentes F, Perez-Diaz D, Sanz-Sanchez M, Martin-Llorente C, Guerrero-Sanz JE. 11 March 2004: the terrorist bomb explosions in Madrid, Spain—an analysis of the logistics, injuries sustained and clinical management of casualties treated at the closest hospital. Crit Care. 2005;9:104–11.
44. Bumbašireviæ M, Lesic A, Mitkovic M, Bumbašireviæ V. Treatment of blast injuries of the extremity. J Am Acad Orthop Surg. 2006;14:77–81.
45. Ad-El DD, Mintz Y, Eldad A, et al. Suicide bombing injuries: the Jerusalem experience of exceptional tissue damage posing a new challenge for the reconstructive surgeons. Plast Reconstr Surg. 2006;118:383–7.
46. Peleg K, Liran A, Tessone A, Givon A, Orenstein A, Haik J. Do burns increase the severity of terror injuries? J Burn Care Res. 2008;29:887–92.
47. Braverman I, Wexler D, Oren M. A novel mode of infection with hepatitis B: penetrating bone fragments due to the explosion of a suicide bomber. Isr Med Assoc J. 2002;4:525–9.
48. Orlac WC, DeBakey ME, Holcomb JB, et al. Mortality from isolated civilian penetrating extremity injury. J Trauma. 2005;59:217–22.
49. The Meir Amit Intelligence and Information Center. Initial findings of the profile of palestinian terrorists who carried out attacks in Israel in the current wave of terrorism. 2015. p. 1–5. http://www.terrorism-info.org.il/en/article/20900. Accessed 7 Jan 2018.
50. Hanoch J, Feigin E, Pikarsky A, et al. Stab wounds associated with terrorist activities in Israel. JAMA. 1996;276:388–90.
51. Reid MJ, Yakeley J. The violent true believer as a "lone wolf"—psychoanalytic perspectives on terrorism. Behav Sci Law. 2014;32:347–65.
52. Almogy G, Kedar A, Bala M. When a vehicle becomes a weapon: intentional vehicular assaults in Israel. Scand J Trauma Resusc Emerg Med. 2016;24:149.
53. Champion HR, Bellamy RF, Roberts CP, Leppaniemi A. A profile of combat injury. J Trauma. 2003;54(5 Suppl):S13–9.
54. Smith ER, Shapiro G, Sarani B. The profile of wounding in civilian public mass shooting fatalities. J Trauma Acute Care Surg. 2016;81:86–92.
55. Kelly RW. Active Shooter: recommendations and analysis for risk mitigation. NYPD Printing Section. https://www1.nyc.gov/assets/nypd/downloads/pdf/counterterrorism/active-shooter-analysis2016.pdf. Accessed 11 Jan 2018.
56. Holcomb JB, Stansbury LG, Champion HR, Wade C, Bellamy RF. Understanding combat casualty care statistics. J Trauma. 2006;60:397–401.
57. Blair JP, Schweit KW. A study of active shooter incidents, 2000-2013. Texas State University and the Federal Bureau of Investigation, US Department of Justice, 2014. https://hazdoc.colorado.edu/bitstream/handle/10590/2712/C022901.pdf?sequence=1. Accessed 12 Jan 2018.
58. Belmont PJ Jr, McCriskin BJ, Sieg RN, Burks R, Schoenfeld AJ. Combat wounds in Iraq and Afghanistan from 2005 to 2009. J Trauma Acute Care Surg. 2012;73:3–12.

The Emergency Room During Mass Casualty Incidents

4

Hany Bahouth

Abbreviations

AD	Administrative director
CEO	Chief executive officer
EMSC	Emergency medical services coordinator
ER	Emergency room
HN	Head nurse
MCI	Mass casualty incident
MedDir	Medical director

4.1 Introduction

Mass casualty incidents (MCIs), man-made or natural, have increased in recent years. In the 1970s, man-made events accounted for 16.5% of disasters and 4.3% of related deaths; in the 1990s, the number rose to 42.0% and 9.5%, respectively (not including "complex emergencies" involving armed conflict and a total breakdown of authority) [1]. There are different types of MCIs, primarily categorized as either progressive disasters or a sudden disaster. A progressive disaster is easier to manage in terms of preparedness and response due to its advancing nature (Hurricane storm). However, a sudden MCI is much more challenging for the entire medical system at local, regional, and national levels. The challenges are organizational, logistical, and relate to a wide range of medical and nonmedical fields through the different pre-hospital and inter-hospital phases of the event, including triage.

H. Bahouth (✉)
Trauma and Emergency Surgery, Rambam Medical Center, Haifa, Israel
e-mail: h_bahouth@rambam.health.gov.il

Y. Kluger et al. (eds.), *WSES Handbook of Mass Casualties Incidents Management*, Hot Topics in Acute Care Surgery and Trauma,
https://doi.org/10.1007/978-3-319-92345-1_4

Successful management of sudden MCIs requires a strong and planned coordination between the medical systems at their different phases of response and between the medical systems and the non-medical systems such as the police department, army, media, communication systems, and other ancillaries.

In most of hospitals around the world, including the Western countries, emergency rooms (ERs) lack the infrastructure to effectively manage an MCI [2]. Emergency rooms are generally designed with sufficient, but not excess, space [3]. Some hospitals are now increasing bed capacity by utilizing hallways, enabling double occupancy in patient rooms, and converting other non-treatment spaces in order to increase their ability to meet patient surges during a disaster [3]. Modular ERs with fold-and-stack walls, curtains, or other structures such as tents can help increase the available treatment spaces during MCIs [3].

Normally, the ER serves as a gateway to the hospital and is the most available point of access to immediate health care, but it also plays a central role during disasters. Pre-event preparedness and extensive early and detailed planning for mass casualty events is crucial to optimize care, to minimize chaos, and to improve outcomes [4].

Activation of an ER plan must be identical, regardless the time of day or day of week, including holidays. All types of hazards must be taken into consideration, and the plan must be able to meet the needs of the four main categories of MCI (conventional, chemical/toxicological, biological, and radiation).

The aim of this chapter is to describe systematically the setup and response of the ER in a MCI, with a specific focus on the logistical and organizational details.

4.2 Emergency Room Response in MCI

The basic actions and activation of the ER for the different types of MCI are similar and share many elements. These basic and common elements include (see Fig. 4.1):

1. Notification and Verification of MCI
2. ER activation
   - ER evacuation
   - Assumption of responsibility by key personnel
   - ER triage setup and implementation
   - Staff deployment
   - Equipment deployment and logistics
   - Setup and organization of ER treatment sites
   - Setup and organization of additional treatment sites
   - Patient identification, registration, and tracking

It should be noted that, as shown in Fig. 4.1, once a decision has been made to activate the ER for the MCI, several parallel processes are activated. All of these processes are discussed below in fuller detail. In addition, there are additional considerations that must be understood well before the MCI. These are discussed in Sect. 4.5.

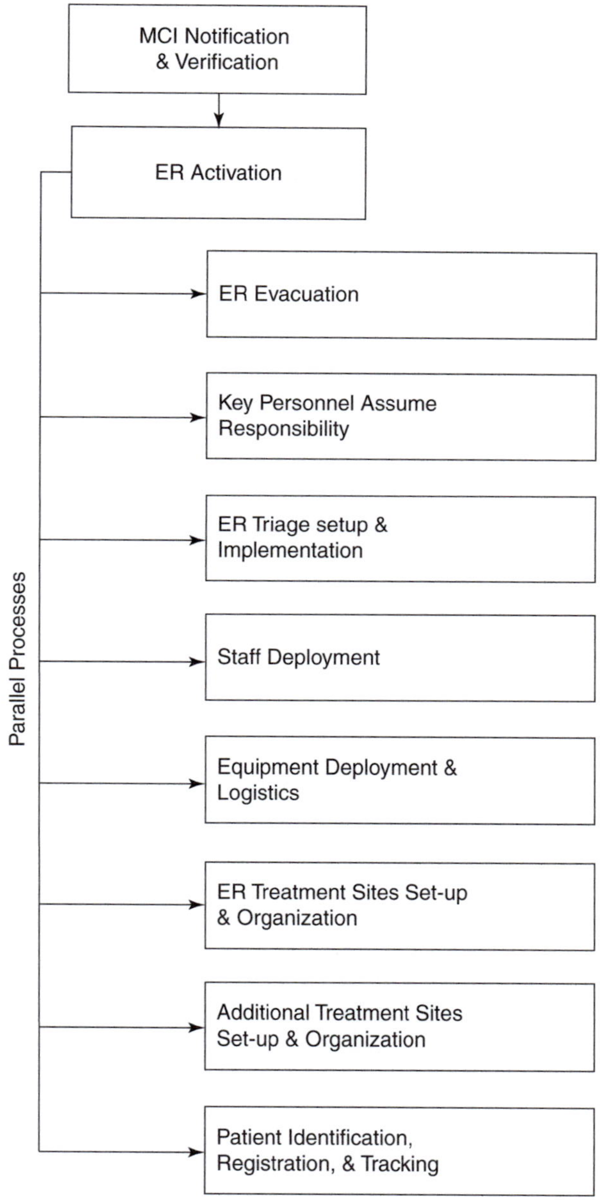

Fig. 4.1 Emergency room response in mass casualty incidents

4.3 Notification and Verification of MCI

Official notification and verification of a MCI must be managed in a simple, organized, and systematic manner based on predefined protocols and checklists. Notification and general awareness that a disastrous event has occurred may come via unofficial channels such as the news, media, or the admission of a patient claiming injury in MCI. Official notification may come through hospital channels (administration, authorized personnel, hospital security) or recognized public services (police, fire department, pre-hospital emergency medical system (EMS)). Hence, the need for verification of the MCI is critical before the ER is activated to implement MCI response plan.

Verification must include information on the type of MCI, its extent, estimated number of injured adults and children, the location of the event, and the expected time for the first patient's arrival.

Immediately upon verification of the MCI, a discussion should be held between the authorized decision-makers, such as the senior surgeon on call, the senior ER physician on call, and the charge nurse for a brief evaluation of the situation, and to confirm officially the decision to activate the ER for the MCI [1].

Approval to activate the ER for the MCI depends on the hospital/local/national policy. Different countries utilize different protocols, with some requiring the formal approval of the hospital's chief executive officer (CEO), director, or his deputy.

The Israeli experience, which has had to manage numerous MCIs, revealed that there was a low threshold for implementation of the MCI protocol due to difficulties in obtaining accurate and detailed information. As a result, the decision was made that a CEO or his/her deputy was required to approve activation of the ER in response to a large-scale event.

4.4 Emergency Room Activation

Activation of the ER in a MCI begins immediately after notification and verification of the event, and the appropriate approval to respond to the event. The responsibilities for activating the ER are divided between designated staff such as the senior surgeon on call, the ER senior physician on call, and/or the ER charge nurse, based on predefined protocols and checklists.

Activation of the ER includes: implementation of in-house and call-in lists; verification of available beds in the ER and alternate care sites; notification of all hospital facilities outside of the ER, including the operating room, blood bank, radiology, laboratory, and hospital security; triage site activation, notification of meeting points for medical staff, activation of the emergency stretcher plan, deployment of equipment and carts, and distribution of identification vests and portable radios.

4.4.1 Evacuation of the Emergency Room

The ER may have only minutes to accommodate the first wave of casualties that may arrive without any warning, quickly overwhelming department resources [5, 6]. The first step in preparation is to clear the ER of non-critical patients, preferably via a central exit. The surgeon in charge and the ER physician will make decisions with regard to those patients who can be safely moved to preplanned alternate care areas, or discharged. This space will serve as a staging area until floor beds are available. Patients from the ER area will be evacuated to available beds in the hospital. If no beds are available, patients will be placed in corridors, under nursing/ medical supervision as needed [7]. Critical patients will await suitably monitored transportation to an appropriate floor. Documentation is limited to registration of personal details (name, ID number, diagnosis, and gender) and their destination, allowing for the rapid transport of 50–80 patients from the ER within 10 min.

4.4.2 Assumption of Responsibility by Key Personnel

Successful MCI management depends on a few key personnel: the medical director (MedDir), the administrative director (AD), the institute's head nurse (HN) [8], and the emergency medical services coordinator (EMSC) [9]. They have been assigned to their roles well before the MCI occurs. They have been specially trained and will work according to predefined protocols.

The MedDir is usually a highly experienced trauma surgeon or a general surgeon equally experienced in trauma. The MedDir receives all pertinent information from the triage officer and the EMSC, such as the location and magnitude of the MCI and the estimated number of victims [8]. The MedDir responsibilities include, at a minimum:

1. Establishing the trauma teams: The most experienced surgeon in each of these teams is its chief and the only team member who reports directly to the MedDir.
2. Establishing smaller teams to yellow treatment site (see Sect. 4.4.6.2) and assigning a senior surgeon to supervise that area.
3. Implementing the appropriate surgical interventions.
4. Prioritizing surgeries at the operating room, the imaging modalities, specially the CT Scan, and the admissions to Intensive Care Units and wards.
5. Briefing the arriving personnel regarding the MCI.

The AD alleviates the burden of administrative issues from the MedDir. Based on the Israeli experience, it is recommended that directors of Emergency Departments be assigned to this position.

The AD's responsibilities include management of all logistics, including prioritizing admissions, use of imaging modalities, and surgical assignments, ensuring all blood bank-related issues and communications with the hospital administration.

The hospital HN responsibilities include: (a) assisting the MD by managing all nursing-related issues; (b) managing transfer of patients out of the ER; (c) directing the nurses recruited from the wards until more ER nurses arrive; and (d) collecting patient status and disposition data, and, determine if special equipment or resources are needed in the ER.

The EMSC is responsible for updating the triage officer on the type of MCI experienced, the location of the MCI, the expected casualty load, and the extent of injuries [8].

4.4.3 Emergency Room Triage Setup and Implementation

Triage is a vital and critical process for managing MCIs [10]. Problems in the quality of triage are expressed in terms of over-triage and under-triage. Over-triage leads to competition for treating the severely injured. Under-triage results in medical error and delays the provision of medically necessary care. Both problems increase the fatality rate among patients who might have potentially survived. During an actual MCI, the triage officer has time for only a rapid glance at each arrival; this brief examination occurs within a matter of seconds. Their decision must rely on a global clinical impression of the patient rather than on physiologic measurements. Many triage methods exist; one very simple method is the "ask-look-feel" method [6, 9].

The first priority for ER activation is preparation of the triage area outside the ER. The triage officers are the first medical professionals to process the MCI victims in the hospital setting. Originally, this responsibility was reserved for the most senior ER surgeon; however, experience has proven that a less qualified surgeon or ER physician can handle it equally well [11]. Preparation of the triage site requires the triage officer's attendance, two ER nurses, and at least two clerks for patient registration and photography. Severity labeling is performed according to the triage officer's decision. Triaged patients must also be given identifying armbands and charts.

The triage site should have a single entry point. Models employing multiple triage points have been shown to scatter resources and add to confusion [5]. The triage site should be comprised of a wide and comfortable area to provide easy access and exit for ambulances, the stretchers, and for the ease of logistics. The stretcher concentration point must be in close proximity to the triage site.

The triage officer must be fully familiar with the basic concepts of the triage process. Physicians able to fulfill this role should be trained and familiarized with the triage protocol process and documentation as part of their duties before the MCI. Selection of a triage officer should take into account the time of the event (morning, evening, or night shifts) to accommodate the in-hospital staff until the arrival of more experienced personnel.

Re-triage is the dynamic process that occurs inside the ER at the different treatment sites. Some of the red patients will be evaluated and re-triaged to either yellow or green and vice versa (see Sect. 4.4.6).

4.4.4 Staff Deployment

Staff deployment for a sudden MCI is of paramount importance to the successful management of the event. The deployment process has two parallel components: (1) staff deployment from within the hospital and (2) the calling in of staff from outside the hospital. Matching the sudden surge of patients with adequate staff in a sudden MCI can affect the level and the quality of care in such events [7].

Staff deployment includes doctors, nurses, radiology technicians, blood bank technicians, laboratory technicians, transport personnel, security staff, and clerks.

4.4.4.1 Staff Deployment Within the Hospital

There are several methods for deploying staff from within the hospital—via a hospital-wide paging system, in-hospital public announcement system and speakers, and/or beepers and cell phones that are automatically activated by a central computer [4]. To allow rapid mobilization of medical teams, a core of nurses who normally work outside the ER should have been trained on a regular basis to work in the ER and to become familiar with its setup and supplies. These volunteer nurses should spend several shifts a year in the ER to retain their knowledge and skills. When a MCI occurs, these "cross-trained" nurses are responsible to immediately report to the ER [4]. In addition, all surgical attending physicians and residents present in the hospital should report to the ER, where the senior administrator on call will assign and direct them to care areas within the ER. Non-general surgical residents from specialties such as gynecology, ENT, and ophthalmology should also report and be utilized as necessary.

4.4.4.2 Staff Deployment from Home

A disaster plan "call tree" must be in place in each department, with an established and well-practiced notification process such as an alphanumeric paging system or cellphones. Hospital administration should have up-to-date staffing lists on hand with telephone numbers and areas of expertise for all personnel [4].

The main weakness of the "call tree" method is the assumption that the listed people are available and will answer their phones [7]. This weakness must be taken into account throughout the deployment process. All staff and personnel who are called in from home need to bring their hospital/institute identification badges or tags to simplify their identification and assignment.

Prearranged meeting points are part of the personnel call-in plan, to facilitate the assignment of recruited staff as needed, according to their specifically assigned roles and to control the "staff overcrowding phenomena" in the ER. The overcrowding of personnel is a true challenge in MCIs and this "mass provider's incident" is well known in such situations. The senior hospital administrator is also responsible for crowd control, turning away curious and unnecessary staff members and bystanders with the help of the security staff [4].

4.4.5 Equipment Deployment and Logistics

Critical to the management of any MCI is the presence and adequate maintenance of medical supplies and equipment. A system for accessing all equipment that may be needed during an MCI, such as mechanical ventilators, tourniquets, regulated medical waste bags, cleaning supplies, and additional resources such as narcotic pain medicine, antibiotics, bags of crystalloid fluid, and intravenous tubing, must have been arranged long before the MCI occurred [12].

A shortage of equipment and medical supplies has been reported in different previous MCIs. Medical supplies located in the basement were destroyed or inaccessible after the Northridge earthquake incident and in the Houston, Texas flooding of 2001 [13]. During the Rhode Island Station Nightclub fire, receiving hospitals quickly ran out of intubation supplies and the supply of antidote was depleted rapidly after the Tokyo sarin gas attack [5].

The ER design must incorporate appropriate storage areas for such items. Given the current trend at medical institutions for small inventories and "just-in-time" supply management, a determination about what is considered "critical" stock and where it should be stored must be made on a per-hospital basis depending on local standards [12, 14].

Available medical supplies and equipment must meet the needs for both conventional and non-conventional MCIs (hazardous materials [HazMat]) and be stored at pre-designed sites. Based on the Israeli experience, it is recommended to store the HazMat equipment for MCIs outside the ER, but in close proximity to the decontamination site, including intubation and resuscitation supplies, wire mesh, a gurneys barricades, and markers.

Ready to use predesigned carts that include the basic equipment for management of injured patients are also recommended. These carts are designed based on the Advanced Trauma Life Support® methodology which uses the A, B, C method (Airway, Breathing, Circulation) to locate all items on any cart, thereby simplifying their use and placement. Special carts are available for conventional and non-conventional MCIs, and pediatric use. All carts should be stored in designated MCI storage rooms in the ER vicinity. In our institute, the expiratory date for the equipment and medications in these carts and storage rooms is controlled by computer software.

Additional logistic considerations include provision of adequate food supplies for the increased staff and patients, planning for sufficient equipment on hand, and ensuring the availability of staff to continuously clean medical instruments and maintain the medical equipment.

4.4.6 Setup and Organization of ER Treatment Sites

The most common setup of the MCI treatment sites is to have three sites, designated as red, yellow, and green.

4.4.6.1 Red Site Treatment Area

The red site is designated for treatment of the severely injured. It can be located in a shock-trauma room (if available) or any other designated area in the ER. Available equipment at this site must meet the need for monitoring (ventilators, cardiac monitors, pulse oximeters) and treating life threatening conditions. If the scale of event is quite large, with more space needed to accommodate the severely injured, preplanned spaces on the same floor and in close proximity to the original red site should be opened. The senior surgeon on call is in charge of this site, with the most senior surgeons and physicians and nurses providing care there. Generally, at least one physician and one nurse should be assigned to each patient at this site. As more help arrives, additional nurse and physicians can then be assigned to this site and to the yellow sites.

4.4.6.2 Yellow Site Treatment Area

The yellow site is designated for treatment of the moderately injured. It too is located in a designated area inside the ER. Preferably, a surgeon should in charge of this site (if available). In unavailable, an ER or other physician can be assigned until the surgeon arrives. Mainly junior surgeons and ER physicians staff this site. One physician and one nurse can take care of more than one injured patient until additional medical staff arrives.

4.4.6.3 Green Site Treatment Area

The green site is designated for treatment of the mildly injured. These patients, often referred to as "walking wounded," typically comprise 50% of MCI victims, and can be managed in an area further removed from the ER. A senior or junior physician may be in charge of this site. It is recommended to provide a minimum of one nurse for every ten patients.

4.4.7 Setup and Organization of Additional Treatment Sites

Additional treatment sites relate to pediatric patients and victims with mental health issues.

4.4.7.1 Pediatric Site

It is recommended that the pediatric site be located within the ER and not in a remote area. Severely injured pediatric patients should be treated at the red site. All others can be treated at a designated pediatric site. The pediatric surgeon on call or the senior pediatric ER physician should be in charge of this site. As mentioned above, carts and equipment should be readily available based on the pre-arranged equipment distribution and logistics plan.

4.4.7.2 Mental Health Site

The mental health site is a designated area for patients with acute stress reactions or other behavioral health problems. A psychiatrist, psychologist, or social worker can be in charge of this site. One nurse for ten patients is recommended.

4.4.8 Patient Identification, Registration, and Tracking

Outside the ER and immediately following triage, every patient must be registered by at least two clerks to prevent bottleneck at the entrance of the ER [15, 16]. During registration, each patient receives a colored armband (red, yellow, green) and medical chart. They should be assigned a temporary identification number that is used as their temporary medical record number (T-number) which is placed on their armband and the medical chart. The color of the armband is used to direct the patient to the appropriate treatment site. The medical chart should have been designed in advance (by the medical and nursing staff) to facilitate simple and basic medical documentation and basic information. As stated above, no written documentation is done at the triage site, only categorization of severity. Digital cameras should be used by one of the registration clerks to photograph comatose or intubated patients and infants, and anyone without an attending family member. The T-number must be included in the picture.

Patient tracking during an MCI is essential, and a real-time assessment of patient location is paramount. This is critical not only for the efficient management of patient flow and resource allocation, including operative suites and ancillary testing, but also for updating families with regard to patient status [17].

Potential patient tracking systems include use of a bar code as well as manual tracking systems. If bar codes are used, computers and bar code scanners should be accessible at all entrances and exits to the ER.

In Israel, a national, manual-input casualty tracking system called "Adam," developed by Rambam Medical Center in Haifa, aids in tracking patients across facilities.

Based on the Israeli experience, fully computerized systems for patient documentation have been found unsuitable for the chaotic MCI environment and paper-based systems that are used during large MCIs are much safer [4].

4.5 Additional Important Considerations

4.5.1 Emergency Room Inter-communication

Communication in the ER throughout the MCI is critical. The communication system used, between all staff involved in the MCI as well as external parties (EMS, polices, etc.), must be available, reliable, clear, and secure. Communication problems and failure have been common in past MCIs and are frequently raised as an issue for improvement in debriefings after the events [18].

Channels for communications must be available to ensure contact from outside the hospital to the hospital and vice versa. This section focuses on ER communication.

Failure of communication inside hospitals can be a result of extensive damage to landlines (earthquake, flooding), damage to cellular towers, overwhelmed cellular lines, and varied signal strength. While cellular telephones are extremely useful, cellular networks have failed in recent MCI scenarios [19, 20]. In such cases, two-way radios can provide a secure and clear alternative. Two-way radios should be maintained on hand in a secure location and be fully charged. If two-way radios are used, at least two channels are needed: one for medical communications and one for security. The medical channel is dedicated for communication between the triage area, operating room, radiology services, transport, treatment sites, command center, and the surgeon on charge of the event. Limiting the number of personell using the two-ways radios will improve the communication process and increase its efficacy.

4.5.2 The "One Way" ER Concept

A concept that is widely implemented in the Israeli ER and states that the flow and movement of the patients into and out of the ER is unidirectional. The main idea behind this concept is to accommodate and maximize efficiency in managing surge volume. The front entrance is utilized solely for patient triage, and the rear exit is used solely for patient egress, creating controlled patient flow through the department. Patient flow should occur from the ER to alternate inpatient destinations (operating room or radiology/testing areas, ICU or ward bed). All patients leaving the ER for the radiology department (mainly CT scan) are admitted to a nearby facility that is staffed by a senior physician and nurse, waiting for medical decision and plan for the final destination of the patient. Minimizing patient movement throughout the hospital during a MCI also helps minimize patient misidentification and confusion.

A "controller" should be at the exit door from the ER. The role of the controller, either a nurse or clerk, is to ensure full documentation in the medical chart and verify the patient's destination.

4.5.3 Response to Chemical, Biological, and Radiation Events

The basic concepts for activating the ER for a conventional or non-conventional MCI are the same. The main difference is the need to protect hospital staff and for decontamination and/or isolation of the injured. Decontamination and isolation facilities must be appropriately located [6]. The response to one of these hazards has to be rapid and occurs prior to entering the ER. Failure of the decontamination process may result in significant hazards to the treating staff members [9, 21, 22]. It is recommended that the decontamination site be close to the ER, in order to make the process easier.

The protocol of the Israel National Committee on HazMat preparedness is as follows: personal protective equipment (PPE) of at least class C or equivalent must be made available to the decontamination staff quickly and in sufficient quantities. Staff in the ER are provided only with respiratory protection and butyl Rubber gloves [14].

Decontamination is carried out with warm water showers and ancillary disrobing and soaping equipment. A hot line is permanently marked on the pavement.

Patient isolation may be required in the event of a biologic or infectious MCI. Hence, the ER must also have a dedicated isolation area with strict protocols for management of these special situations.

4.5.4 Diagnostics and Blood Tests

There are a few considerations to be noted with regard to blood tests, X-rays, and ultrasonography during MCI.

Two blood tests are recommended in MCIs: (1) blood typing and crossmatching; (2) arterial blood gases. Based on the Israel experience, it is recommended to be very selective in taking blood for lab tests. Note that patients with a "red" designation will need many more tests; those with a "yellow" or "green" designation should have blood tests taken only as needed.

Chest and pelvic X-ray studies should be requested strictly based on need. The main issue regarding these types of X-rays within the ER is the movement of staff outside the room or behind a wall, unless the space is divided by walls and each injured patient is treated in separate room.

Our and others experience during MCIs indicates that bedside diagnostic ultrasonography is an excellent tool to further triage in the ER of hemodynamically unstable patients, internal torso injury in comatose patients, or in patients who have external signs of torso penetration from blast shrapnel [23, 24].

4.6 Summary

Handling mass casualty incidents is always highly challenging in terms of organization, logistics, and medical aspects. Optimizing the response to any MCI requires great efforts at the local, regional, and national levels, and well-organized coordination between different aspects and phases of management and between different authorities. At the hospital level, the setup and response of the emergency room plays a crucial rule in MCIs. This ER response includes many parallel processes to activate and prepare the ER for handling and managing the casualties of the event. As described in this chapter, the overall process must be well organized and controlled to achieve best results and efficiency. The process itself is based on many organizational details, as described, and on MCI-specific altered standards of care that are unfamiliar to the staff. Utilizing the same methodologies as in routine emergencies is doomed to failure. Predefined protocols will have a major positive effect on the entire process. An effective method for testing efficacy of protocols and to identify weaknesses is through repeated drills of the ER staff, including both the medical and non-medical teams. By becoming familiar with the protocols and the details of the entire MCI response process, the ER staff will avoid the phenomena of "Paper Plan Syndrome," and the teams will become much more confident and effective when working in the emergency room under the constraints of a mass casualty incident.

References

1. World Health Organization (WHO). Mass casualty management systems: strategies and guidelines for building health sector capacity. Health Action in Crises Injury and Violence Prevention. Geneva: WHO; April 2007. http://www.who.int/hac/techguidance/tools/mcm_guidelines_en.pdf.
2. Niska RW, Shimizu IM. Hospital preparedness for emergency response: United States, 2008. Natl Health Stat Report. 2011;37:1–14.
3. Woolard RH, Borron SW, Mackay JM. Chapter 21: Emergency department design. In: Ciottone GR, editor. Ciottone's disaster medicine. Philadelphia: Elsevier. p. 125–9.

4. Singer AJ, Singer AH, Halperin P, Kaspi G, Assaf J. Medical lessons learned from terror attacks in Israel. J Emerg Med. 2007;32(1):87–92.
5. Okumura T, Suzuki K, Fukuda A, Kohama A, Takasu N, Ishimatsu S, Hinohara S. The Tokyo subway sarin attack: disaster management, Part 1: community emergency response. Acad Emerg Med. 1998;5(6):613–7.
6. Almogy G, Belzberg H, Mintz Y, Pikarsky AK, Zamir G, Rivkind AI. Suicide bombing attacks: update and modifications to the protocol. Ann Surg. 2004;239(3):295–303.
7. Lynn M. Mass casualty incidents: the nuts and bolts of preparedness and response for acute disasters. New York: Springer Science + Business Media; 2016.
8. Sofer D, Klausner JM. Trauma system configurations in other countries: the Israeli model. Surg Clin North Am. 2012;92(4):1025–40.
9. Kluger Y, Mayo A, Soffer D, Adadgem D, Halperin P. Functions and principles in the management of bombing mass casualty incidents: lessons learned at the Tel-Aviv Souraski Medical Center. Eur J Emerg Med. 2004;11(6):329–34.
10. Foley E, Reisner AT. Chapter 54: Triage. In: Ciottone GR, editor. Disaster medicine. Philadelphia: Elsevier Health Sciences; 2006. p. 337–43.
11. Cushman G, Pachter HL, Beaton HL. Two New York City hospitals' surgical response to the September 11, 2001, terrorist attack in New York City. J Trauma. 2003;54(1):147–55.
12. Gale SC, Donovan CM, Tinti M, Ahmed H, Gracias VH. Organization and operations management at the health care facility. Ann Emerg Med. 2017;69(1S):S29–35.
13. Nates JL. Combined external and internal hospital disaster: impact and response in a Houston trauma center intensive care unit. Crit Care Med. 2004;32(3):686–90.
14. Halpern P, Goldberg SA, Keng JG, Koenig KL. Principles of Emergency Department facility design for optimal management of mass-casualty incidents. Prehosp Disaster Med. 2012;27(2):204–12.
15. Benson M, Koenig KL, Schultz CH. Disaster triage: START, then SAVE—a new method of dynamic triage for victims of a catastrophic earthquake. Prehosp Disaster Med. 1996;11(2):117–24.
16. Feliciano DV, Anderson GV Jr, Rozycki GS, Ingram WL, Ansley JP, Namias N, Salomone JP, Cantwell JD. Management of casualties from the bombing at the Centennial Olympics. Am J Surg. 1998;176(6):538–43.
17. Vanderwagen C. Implementing the National Health Security Strategy [White paper]. Aptean website. http://www.irms360.com/vanderwagen-national-health-security-strategy. Accessed 28 Apr 2018.
18. D'Andrea SM, Goralnick E, Kayden SR. 2013 Boston Marathon bombings: overview of an emergency department response to a mass casualty incident. Disaster Med Public Health Prep. 2013;7(2):118–21.
19. Kirschenbaum L, Keene A, O'Neill P, Westfal R, Astiz ME. The experience at St Vincent's Hospital, Manhattan, on September 11, 2001: preparedness, response, and lessons learned. Crit Care Med. 2005;33(1 Suppl):S48–52.
20. Gavagan TF, Smart K, Palacio H, Dyer C, Greenberg S, Sirbaugh P, Fishkind A, Hamilton D, Shah U, Masi G, Ivey RT, Jones J, Chiou-Tan FY, Bloodworth D, Hyman D, Whigham C, Pavlik V, Feigin RD, Mattox K. Hurricane Katrina: medical response at the Houston Astrodome/Reliant Center Complex. South Med J. 2006;99(9):933–9.
21. Horton DK, Orr M, Tsongas T, Leiker R, Kapil V. Secondary contamination of medical personnel, equipment and facilities resulting from hazardous materials events, 2003-2006. Disaster Med Public Health Prep. 2008;2(2):104–13.
22. Centers for Disease Control Prevention (CDC). Update: investigation of bioterrorism-related anthrax and interim guidelines for exposure management and antimicrobial therapy, October 2001. MMWR Morb Mortal Wkly Rep. 2001;50(42):909–19.
23. Sajed D. The history of point-of-care ultrasound use in disaster and mass casualty incidents. Virtual Mentor. 2010;12:744–9.
24. Sztajnkrycer MD, Baez AA, Luke A. FAST ultrasound as an adjunct to triage using the START mass casualty triage system: a preliminary descriptive system. Prehosp Emerg Care. 2006;10:96–102.

Triage and Clinical Evaluation in MCI

5

Yoram Klein

5.1 Introduction

Clinical evaluation is one of the fundamental elements of medicine. There are several factors in mass casualty incident (MCI) that make clinical evaluation more challenging. In the first phase of the management of the patient in MCI, all clinical evaluations should be done in a triage mode. That means, the diagnostic efforts should be focused on identifying immediate life-threatening conditions and quick decision about where the patient should be transferred to, in the next stage. The nature of the incidents allows very short time for these tasks. Another important aspect is the fact that in large-scale incidents the availability of ancillary diagnostic modalities is limited. Due to the anticipated discrepancy between number of patients and the availability of medical professionals from relevant specialty, many times less experienced caregivers, sometimes even from unrelated disciplines, are expected to evaluate and manage complicated trauma patients.

In summary, the principles of the clinical guidelines for MCI, should reflect these challenges, and provide tools for the average caregiver, from a non-trauma related specialty, for quick and safe evaluation of the patient with minimal use of laboratory or imaging studies.

Y. Klein (✉)
Trauma and Critical Care Division, Department of Surgery, Sheba Medical Center, Ramat-Gan, Israel
e-mail: Yoram.klein@sheba.health.gov.il

Y. Kluger et al. (eds.), *WSES Handbook of Mass Casualties Incidents Management*, Hot Topics in Acute Care Surgery and Trauma,
https://doi.org/10.1007/978-3-319-92345-1_5

5.2 Triage

The definition of triage is sorting the patients in MCI according to their medical needs and available resources [1]. Triage is the most characteristic medical activity during MCI. There are multiple levels of triage during MCI. The first is the field medical triage. The principle is simple, the paramedic in the field should decide whether the patient should receive immediate treatment, immediate transfer, or delayed management. There is no universal set of rules that dictate which patient should belong to what option. The most accepted mode of clinical triage is the simple triage and rapid treatment (START) method. The caregiver is expected to rapidly evaluate the patient's ability to walk, his level of consciousness, hemodynamic status, and respiratory efforts within 1 min [2, 3]. Usually, available resources such as number of ambulances, number of caregivers, available air evacuation, and the distance from the hospital will determine the extent of the medical treatment in the field and the speed of evacuation. In areas with advanced emergency services, the minimal acceptable treatment in the field is securing airway patency, improving oxygenation with supplemental oxygen, mechanical ventilation or needle drainage of tension pneumothorax, and control of external bleeding, which is probably the most important prehospital intervention to avoid preventable death [4].

The second level of triage is the destination triage. Primary destination triage means sending the patient from the field directly to the proper hospital according to the injury pattern and receiving hospital capabilities. Secondary triage means sending the patient to the nearest hospital regardless of the specific injuries and receiving hospital capabilities. The first triage mode is probably the most efficient mode of triage that allow the shortest time to definitive care. Secondary triage is the mode of choice in case where there is shortage of ambulances that dictate repeated short rounds of the ambulances [5]. Availability of helicopters sometimes allows sending stable patients to remote hospitals in order to avoid overwhelming the local facilities.

5.3 Clinical Evaluation and Triage in the Hospital

The first triage in the hospital is at the entrance to the emergency department. The only purpose of this process is to send the patient to the right admission site. The triage post at the entrance is notorious to be a potential bottle neck in the flow of victims into the hospital. In order to avoid this, the decision must be made very quickly. It is based on a brief visual of the patient focusing on respiratory movement, estimation of skin perfusion (color, temperature, and moisture), hemodynamic estimation based on the quality of the radial pulse, and significant external bleeding. The level of consciousness should be estimated based on purposeful movements. No other clinical activities should be done at this site. In most centers, the patients are divided between four admission sites: patients with respiratory, hemodynamic, or level of consciousness impairment should be triaged to the critical site; patients on stretchers will go to moderate-severe site; mobile patients with minimal injuries will be sent to the walking patients site; and patients with no signs of injury but with obvious acute stress reaction will be sent to emotional stress site.

After admission of the patient to the site, the medical team will evaluate and stabilize the patient according to the advanced trauma life support (ATLS) principles. Like in the pre-hospital scene, the physician should decide whether the patient needs immediate intervention (definitive airway procedure, thoracic drainage for tension pneumothorax, external bleeding control, etc.), immediate operation (e.g., a patient with low blood pressure and penetrating abdominal injury), or they can be delayed for further workup. There are few factors that need to be considered regarding the management of the trauma patient during MCI. The basic principle of MCI is not to divide the resources between the patients. The efforts should be focused on finding the salvageable patients, that will be significantly harmed from delaying treatment, and concentrate the resources on them. In large-scale incidents, every medical team will have to simultaneously manage more than one patient. It means that the team leader will have to rapidly determine the severity of the patient's condition in the primary survey and focus most of the efforts on the most severe patients. Some routines must be modified during MCI in order to adjust to resources limited environment. For example, if blood sample for type and cross will be indiscriminately sent for every patient, the blood bank technicians will be overwhelmed by the load and there is a risk that blood products supply for patients in hemorrhagic shock will be delayed. So, during MCI blood sample for type and cross should be sent only for patients with suspected bleeding [6].

The next level of triage is prioritizing patients that need limited resources. The first one is selecting patients that need urgent operations. Four categories of surgeries can be identified. Priority 1 operations include procedures for hemorrhage control or evacuation of intracranial extra-axial hematoma with imminent herniation. Priority 2 includes procedures for ischemic limbs. Priority 3 are procedures for control of contamination (i.e., hemodynamic normal patients with suspected bowel injury or patients suffering from open fractures of long bones). Priority 4 includes all other operations. Patients with priority 1 indication will be transferred to the OR immediately upon establishing the indication for surgery. The rest will be prioritized for surgery according to the clinical judgment of the attending surgeon, based on available surgical teams, operation theatres, and whether more victims are expected to arrive to the hospital [7].

Imaging studies are subjected to triage as well. Extended focus abdominal sonography for trauma (e-Fast) had revolutionized trauma management in the past decades. An ultrasound device should be available in the admission sites. Its value as a screening tool for thoracic abdomen and even extremity injuries is well established [8]. No mobile X-ray should be done in the admission sites. The most important imaging study is the CT scan, which is naturally a limited resource. Up to 6–7 patients per hour can be scanned using a trauma protocol [9]. The first priority for the CT are patients with head injuries and impaired level of consciousness. Next are other severely injured patients, after respiratory and hemodynamic stabilization that need further imaging. The third priority are vascular imaging studies for suspected ischemic limbs. The rest of the patients that need other imaging studies should be prioritized individually, according to their specific needs [10].

In most hospitals, the most limited resource is available intensive care beds. Unlike beds in the emergency department that can be quickly cleared by discharging most of the patients either home or to other departments, beds in the ICU are usually occupied by critically ill patients that can't be discharged. This fact together with the documented over-triage to the ICU demand careful planning for creation of options for extending the ICU surge capacity of the hospital. Strict criteria for triage patients to the ICU during MCI should be implemented. The triage process for the ICU should be done by senior physician, preferably the trauma director or an attending ICU physician [11].

5.4 Summary

Logistic organizing and commanding issues were always considered the most problematic aspects of MCI. But, more than everything, this is an extreme clinical challenge. In this situation, less experienced providers might need to manage severely injured patients, suffering from injuries due to rare mechanism in civilian hospitals (explosion-related trauma). More than that, they have to adjust to a resource-limited environment, so they have to consider the presence of other victims in their decision making process. The triage process is not a single event in the treatment chain, but rather a repeated, continuous multiple level process. These considerations should be included in every hospital's preparedness, education, and training plans for MCI.

References

1. Robertson-Steel I. Evolution of triage systems. Emerg Med J. 2006;23(2):154–5.
2. Kahn CA, Schultz CH, Miller KT, et al. Does START triage work? An outcomes assessment after a disaster. Ann Emerg Med. 2009;54(3):424–30.
3. Arquilla B, Paladino L, Reich C, Brandler E, Lucchesi M, Shetty S. Using a joint triage model for multi-hospital response to a mass casualty incident in New York City. J Emerg Trauma Shock. 2009;2(2):114–6.
4. Eastridge BJ, Mabry RL, Seguin P, et al. Death on the battlefield (2001–2011): implications for the future of combat casualty care. J Trauma Acute Care Surg. 2012;73(6 Suppl 5):S431–7.
5. Dean MD, Nair SK. Mass-casualty triage: distribution of victims to multiple hospitals using the SAVE model. Eur J Oper Res. 2014;238(1):363–73.
6. Bala M, Kaufman T, Keidar A, et al. Defining the need for blood and blood products transfusion following suicide bombing attacks on a civilian population: a level I single-centre experience. Injury. 2014;45:50–5.
7. Hirshberg A, Stein M, Walden R. Surgical resource utilization in urban terrorist bombing: a computer simulation. J Trauma. 1999;47:545–50.
8. Wydo SM, Seamon MJ, Melanson SW, Thomas P, Bahner DP, Stawicki SP. Portable ultrasound in disaster triage: a focused review. Eur J Trauma Emerg Surg. 2016;42(2):151–9. Epub 2015 Feb 11.

9. Mueck FG, Wirth K, Muggenthaler M, Kreimeier U, Geyer L, Kanz KG, Linsenmaier U, Wirth S. Radiological mass casualty incident (MCI) workflow analysis: single-centre data of a mid-scale exercise. Br J Radiol. 2016;89:20150918.
10. Kluger Y, Mayo A, Soffer D, Aladgem D, Halperin P. Functions and principles in the management of bombing mass casualty incidents: lessons learned at the Tel-Aviv Souraski Medical Center. Eur J Emerg Med. 2004;11:329–34.
11. Lipsky AM, Klein Y, Givon A, Klein M, Hammond JS, Peleg K, Israeli Trauma Group (ITG). Accuracy of initial critical care triage decisions in blast versus non-blast trauma. Disaster Med Public Health Prep. 2014;8(4):326–32.

Providing Information During Mass Casualty Incidents: Information Center, Family-Centered Care and Media Coverage

6

Roni Gagin, Neta HaGani, and David Ratner

6.1 Part I. Operating an Information Center During a Mass Casualty Incident (MCI)

6.1.1 Background

In recent years, there has been an increase in mass casualty incidents (MCIs) that lead to physical, economic, emotional, and social damages [1]. With the increased number of terrorist attacks and unexpected natural disasters worldwide, the entire population is exposed to these events and is potentially at risk of getting hurt [2]. Due to television and social media, reports on MCIs are widespread and have an impact globally. Those who were affected by an MCI use social media platforms to express their needs and to ask for help. Organizations for disaster relief also use social media in order to identify people in need and respond through donations and special delegations of doctors and health professionals [3]. Nowadays, it is essential that every country and local authority will have a set of guidelines for MCIs. Guidelines may differ according to the type of the MCI (natural disasters, terror attacks, etc.) or according to the amount of available resources authorities have [4].

The purpose of this part is to describe a practical model for treating patients and families in hospitals during the first hours of an MCI. This chapter is derived from the field work of the authors during MCIs and according to models and theories in the field of trauma and recovery. We discuss three main issues: (1) MCIs as traumatic events, (2) family support, and (3) a model of an information center for MCIs.

R. Gagin (✉) · N. HaGani
The Social Work Department, Rambam Health Care Campus, Haifa, Israel
e-mail: r_gagin@rambam.health.gov.il; n_hagani@rambam.health.gov.il

D. Ratner
The Spokesman's Office and Public Affairs, Rambam Health Care Campus, Haifa, Israel
e-mail: d_ratner@rambam.health.gov.il

Y. Kluger et al. (eds.), *WSES Handbook of Mass Casualties Incidents Management*, Hot Topics in Acute Care Surgery and Trauma,
https://doi.org/10.1007/978-3-319-92345-1_6

MCIs are considered to be "*traumatic events*." They include a life-threatening experience and serious physical or emotional injury [4]. Traumatic events have personal, social, cultural, and political components, and therefore, the reaction to them varies. Some people might experience different symptoms after a traumatic event like intrusive thoughts, flashbacks, psychological distress, etc. [5]. The most extreme form of these symptoms is the posttraumatic stress disorder (PTSD) [6].

During MCIs, the hospital staff face several professional and personal challenges. First, the discrepancy created between the patient load and the available resources makes it difficult to give high-quality trauma care [7]. Second, working under uncertainty creates a need to adapt quickly and to find alternative solutions to unpredictable problems. These alterations include finding an alternative care site in the waiting areas and allocating equipment, supply, and personnel in a nontraditional way in order to save as many lives as possible [8]. Third, the hospital staff have to treat patients while at the same time they are vulnerable themselves to being hurt and are concerned about their own families. They are required to leave their loved ones behind and report for duty as health professionals. Reluctance to report for work may influence the capacity of the hospital to meet the needs of the population during an MCI [9].

Another challenge is the indirect trauma from exposure to patients who have experienced traumatic events. Clinical research shows that consequences of traumatic events are not restricted to the injured and may affect those around them as well, including family, friends, or healthcare workers [10]. Healthcare workers may experience symptoms like intrusive secondary trauma-related thoughts or memories (flashbacks), avoidance behaviors, sleep disturbances, irritability, and dissociation [11, 12].

6.1.2 Family Support During MCI

Treating the injured and saving lives are the highest priorities during an MCI. However, another important priority is assisting the families of the injured. Immediately with the media reports of a terrorist attack, tens of relatives come to the hospital, looking for missing family members [13]. Since patients belong to their families, it is important to give accurate information and support not only to patients but also to their families. These families are usually in shock, confused, and in a traumatic state [14]. During an MCI, emergency rooms are flooded with concerned family members. The purpose of the family support unit is to be a connecting link between physicians and families, so that physicians can concentrate on helping the injured while family members are taking care of.

Family-centered care is an important element of working with the injured during MCIs. It is based on studies that show that patients' family members play an important role in recovery by providing emotional, social, and functional support. Family-centered care is defined as a mutually beneficial partnership between healthcare providers, patients, and their families [15]. Providing efficient interventions for families of casualties in an MCI may reduce the long-term effect of the trauma. Families are an important source of support for patients from the time of the injury and after they recover. They also play a crucial role during hospitalization in providing information and insight regarding the patient's condition and the patient's physical and emotional resources. Research shows that patients who have strong family and social connections have a faster recovery process, are more compliant with treatment, and have a lower rate of rehospitalization [16, 17].

Family members are facing with anxiety, ambiguity, and uncertainty in the first minutes of receiving the news that their loved ones may have been injured or killed in an incident. They move from hope to despair, crave information, and may become anxious, fearful, and overwhelmed. These moments are the core of the crisis when help is most needed. The intervention is based on principles and guidelines of crisis intervention like providing immediate support, giving maximum information and assistance for immediate problems [14]. It is crucial to have family support service that operates as soon as the MCI occurs in order to provide immediate intervention with relatives in the first minutes and hours of the event. Trained professionals are familiar in the principles of psychological trauma, crisis intervention procedures, victim identification, and support for relatives of MCI victims [13].

6.1.3 Information Center

Information centers in hospitals are created for emergency situations like mass injuries and are meant to give information and crisis intervention to the public during emergency situations. The information center is operated by the social work department in the hospital with cooperation from law enforcement agencies. It works according to specific principles and guidelines of crisis intervention. The first priority is saving lives. The information center operates on several units: (1) the telephone unit, (2) in-hospital information center, (3) families' waiting room, (4) ER, intensive care unit and operating room, and (5) unidentified patients. The main goal of the information center is to provide accurate and reliable information. Other aims include giving support to the families of the injured, assisting families in locating their loved ones and give them information regarding their condition, responding to families' immediate needs, preparing families to meeting their loved ones who got injured or died, providing psychosocial treatment to the injured, and preparing a discharge plan and follow-up plan for rehabilitation.

When an MCI occurs, the hospital notifies the staff. Staff are obligated to report to the hospital after receiving the message either from the hospital or through the media. The information center is opened by the social workers immediately (within 30 min of receiving the news). The telephone unit is the first to be opened. The telephone numbers are announced in the media by the spokesperson, and phone calls from concerned family members of people who might have been affected by the emergency are received (the telephone system used for the information center is based on a different platform than regular telephone lines in order to ensure a stable connection throughout the incident and in cases of total crashing of telephone and cellular lines).

Information regarding casualties comes through a centralized software system built specifically for mass casualty incidents, from the hospital's emergency room and from other hospitals. Data are received through both written and photographed records for those who are unable to give information themselves (unidentified). The information is transferred to the Ministry of Health and local authorities. Employees practice using the computer system twice a year in order to make sure the center operators are well-trained with the online system and are prepared for emergency situations. Also, the staff exercise pen and paper information transference in case of computer or electricity shutdowns.

The information center has several important roles beyond providing information about injured patients through the telephone unit. The first is to serve as an in-hospital information center. Patients and families arriving at the hospital need guidance and support. After locating the patient who the family is looking for, the social workers in the information center accompany the families and prepare them for meeting their loved one, who might be in a severe medical condition.

The second is preparing a family waiting room for families of the injured who arrive at the hospital. In the waiting room, hospital social workers offer a response to immediate needs (food, water) and help with arranging care for small children or elderly relatives who were left behind, with the assistance of the authorities in the community. Family members receive firsthand crisis intervention and are given information regarding patients' treatment progress. Social workers also operate inside the emergency room and intensive care units in the hospital in order to connect between patients and families and help bridge between patients and families and the medical staff. Family members also receive guidance regarding how to handle the media approaching them and asking them for updates about the injured.

The structure of the information center is described in Fig. 6.1:

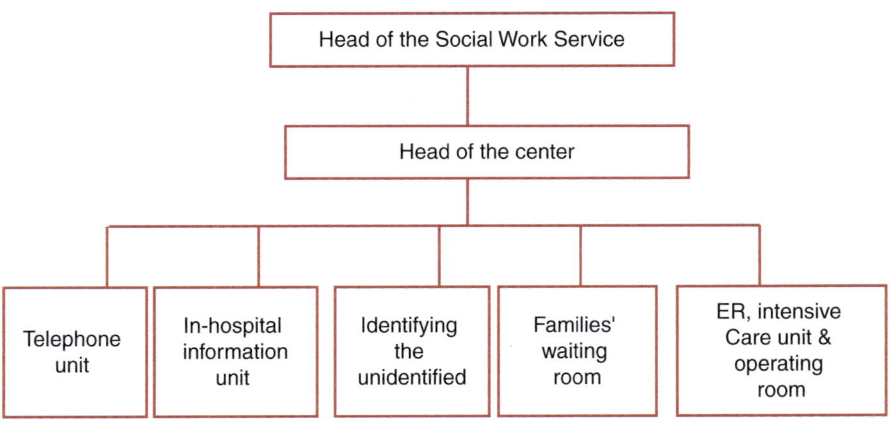

Fig. 6.1 The structure of an information center (Gagin, Cohen & Peled-Avram, 2005)

6.1.3.1 Factors Influencing Information Center Function and Staffing

There are many factors influencing the function of the information center: number of injured, number of unidentified, number of dead, severity of injuries, number of people searching for injured, time of MCI (morning, evening, weekend), and dispersion of injured among hospitals. An MCI may include hundreds or even thousands of injured. Therefore, the information center needs to adjust its staffing and function to different types of MCIs. A wide range MCI may require a larger number of staff and volunteers and a more advanced system for information transferring—for example, large computer screens that present data from all hospitals regarding injured from the incident. In addition, cooperation with the local authorities is sometimes needed in order to take the pressure off the hospitals when the casualty number is very high. The local authorities may assist in relieving the burden by opening a general information center with data regarding patients from different medical centers. When families arrive at the hospital to search for their loved ones, they may be frantic, hysterical, and upset. They might disrupt the medical staff who are treating the injured. Therefore, systems like big screens or other information centers outside of the hospital may assist in handling families in a manner that does not disrupt hospital staff.

The function of the information center also depends on the time of the MCI. During mornings, the hospital is usually fully staffed and it is easier for staff to organize the different units inside the information center. In the middle of the night, it might take longer for staff to arrive at the hospital, especially if the MCI caused traffic jams.

6.1.4 Unidentified Patients

Another important role of the information center during an emergency is identifying unidentified patients with the help of their families. Unidentified patients are injured people who are unable to provide any information regarding their identity. They include patients who are unconscious, injured that passed away at the hospital, injured suffering from shock or severe emotional reaction, babies, or young children. Deceased patients from the scene do not arrive at the hospital but to the forensic institute. At arrival, the unidentified patients are photographed with a digital camera, and the photos are transferred by a computerized system to the information center. Social workers collect personal details and unique signs about the injured from families, medical staff (using forms), and with the help of the Division of Identification and Forensic Science of the police. Cooperation with the Division of Identification and Forensic Science is essential, especially in cases where family members believe an injured patient to be their relative, but the identification is not completely certain, and further information is needed in order to conclusively identify the patient.

The identification process is extremely challenging. Personal belongings (clothes, jewelry) are stripped from injured patients in order to give urgent medical treatment. External appearance may be extremely altered due to injuries (swelling, burns) and medical equipment, blurring individual differences. In addition, family members of the victims may be in deep distress and have difficulties functioning under stress. They may have difficulty identifying the family member. The identification process is a very difficult and emotional process for the family and for the hospital staff. It is intense and filled with uncertainty, confusion, and hope. It is sometimes a long process filled with discrepancy between the sources of information and horrific scenes of the injured. Social workers are there to support families during the process of identification and after.

The information center is officially closed when all immediate needs of the patients and their families have been taken care of and phones calls are no longer coming in. All family members have been matched with patients and the injured have been identified. At that point, social workers are supporting the families of patients who are still missing and preparing them for the high probability of a loss of a loved one. These families are then referred to the forensic institute for identification of the body.

During the MCI and after, the information center cooperates with services in the community like the local municipality, medical centers or clinics, social services, the police and armed forces, in order to provide information during the crisis event and to keep the therapeutic sequence of patients after the crisis is over. Studies conducted in different countries examine the importance of collaboration with authorities and organizations in the community and found that lack of coordination with different community agencies may hinder prevention and response mechanisms [8, 18].

The information center is also there to assist hospital staff and give firsthand treatment for emotional reactions. Hospital staff are exposed to the effects of the crisis via their patients. They are exposed to difficult sights such as injuries, blood, and death. Being a witness to a trauma may lead to secondary trauma among medical and paramedical workers. Therefore, it is important to make sure that the staff are well prepared, through performing emergency drills and by giving emergency training and debriefing.

After the event is over, a debriefing session with the information center staff is conducted which includes providing positive feedback and appreciation, going over the event, determining a treatment plan for injured who were hospitalized, processing staff's emotional reactions to the event, and drawing conclusions regarding the event and future events.

Conclusions

The purpose of this chapter was to present a unique model of working with patients and families during MCIs. This model is based on bio-psycho-social theories and on the accumulated experience and knowledge of hospital staff regarding treatment methods when dealing with victims and their relatives. This model evolves constantly with experiences of different MCIs and with technological developments that allow more efficient ways of distributing information.

One of the crucial elements during crisis intervention is to provide reliable and updated information throughout the event for family members who are confused and filled with uncertainties. The intervention should be adjusted according to hospitalization timeline: from admission, through the hospitalization period and the discharge planning. Follow-up after patients who have been through trauma is important for the therapeutic sequence and in order to ensure the patients' and families' well-being. Follow-up after hospitalization is part of a patient-centered care and has been found to be a contributing factor for preventing rehospitalization, increased adherence to medication and treatment protocols and to patients' satisfaction, among different study populations [19, 20].

Although every MCI has its unique features, it is important to structure work procedures and regulations in the treatment of the families as an essential part of crisis intervention. In addition, exercising these regulations twice a year among staffs is extremely important to validate the level of readiness and hospital's ability to function in real-time MCIs. The separation between medical centers and services in the community needs to be bridged in preparation for mass casualty incidents. In order to increase their preparedness for mass casualty incidents, hospitals should implement community-level planning in the form of guidelines for collaboration with outside organizations like the fire department and law enforcement agencies [8].

Dealing with MCI victims and their relatives may have an effect on healthcare professionals. They may experience a range of feelings like grief, sadness, helplessness, frustration, and fear. Overtime, these symptoms may lead to secondary traumatization or compassion fatigue, especially if the exposure is reoccurring over and over [21]. During MCIs, hospital staff are part of the community who is under an attack. They share the trauma of the victims they treat. This exposes them to extreme personal and professional risks [22]. Therefore, special interventions are needed in order to prevent and to minimize the effect of the shared trauma. These interventions include support groups, debriefing, supervision, and workshops [13].

The first part of this chapter described how medical centers are treating patients and families during the first hours of an MCI and how they handle distributing information to the public. The second part of this chapter describes how medical centers handle media coverage through the experience of medical centers in Israel.

6.2 Part II. Media Coverage During MCI: The Israeli Experience

The speed that news travel in Israel, even discreet or security affiliated news, and the implication on the health system during mass casualty situation is an Israeli phenomenon: in Israel, the presence of media outlets during emergency events is extremely dominant inside hospitals.

Media coverage of mass casualty incidents (MCIs) is quite different from coverage during times of calm. This is particularly so with regard to coverage of hospital-related occurrences that translate into news. In fact, it is reasonable to say that all media coverage in Israeli hospitals during MCI is markedly different from such coverage in many countries.

In order to understand the relationship between media and healthcare systems in Israel, in general, but particularly during MCI, one needs to understand the various parameters that have created unique relationship between the media and hospitals in Israel.

1. In Israel, as in most democracies, the media is free and very competitive. The only restrictions on Israeli media relate to military security issues and patient privacy.
2. Military censorship is used in cases where dissemination of information could in some way negatively affect the nation's security [23]. For example, if an MCI involves soldiers, the media will be instructed by the military censor to refrain from reporting on soldiers if such information could further endanger the soldiers, if the incident itself was classified, and/or until the families of the involved or injured soldiers can be notified.
3. All hospitals in Israel that treat civilian or military victims of trauma and MCI are public hospitals. Thus, it is difficult to prevent journalists from entering publically accessible areas of these hospitals. It is true that there are legal restrictions on the media which arise from patient privacy laws (restrictions which prohibit revealing identifiable patient details without the patient's consent)—but during MCI—those restrictions are less observed by journalists.
4. Geographically, Israel is a very small country where smartphone and internet usage is one of the highest in the world [24].

The ease of accessibility to public hospitals combined with the vast access (by nearly 90% of the population) to smartphones and social networks has created a reality in which every MCI, whether civilian incident or occurring in a "remote" military area, will be reported immediately and widely. Israel is a country where it is almost impossible to "silence" an incident or delay its reporting. As a result, from the moment a rumor of an MCI is released, every hospital in Israel knows that within minutes journalists will be entering the hospital to cover the arrival and treatment of the wounded.

The phenomenon of live onsite broadcasts from within hospitals started during the Second Lebanon War (2006). Not only was there live coverage of the missiles landing in civilian areas, the media setup improvised studios **inside** public hospital areas. This enabled them to broadcast live coverage of the arrival of wounded civilians and soldiers in helicopters or ambulances (Fig. 6.2).

From time to time, there has been discussion as to whether or not media hospital coverage can be stopped or curtailed during MCI, when journalists circulate near emergency rooms, helicopter landing pads, the entrance to hospital departments, and more. This discussion must now consider another component that has made it almost impossible to "hermetically seal" Israeli public hospitals from the media: the broad use of smartphones by Israelis in general.

Smartphones have helped remove the "technological limitations" of live coverage. Every professional or amateur journalist owns a sophisticated camera which is able to transmit live from anywhere and everywhere. In a rare case, when a

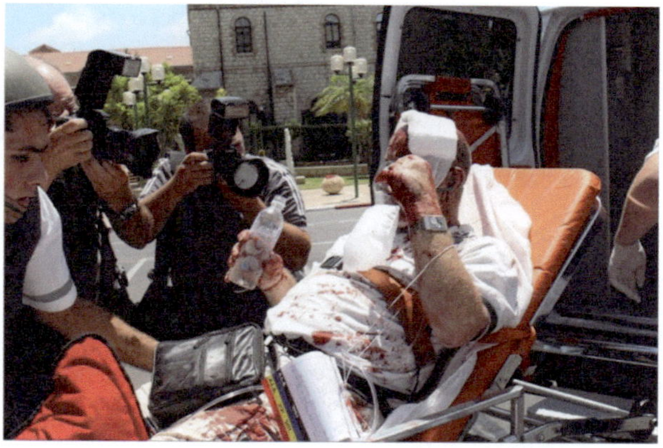

Fig. 6.2 Media photographers during Second Lebanon War (2006) at Rambam hospital in Israel (photo: Pioter Fliter, RHCC)

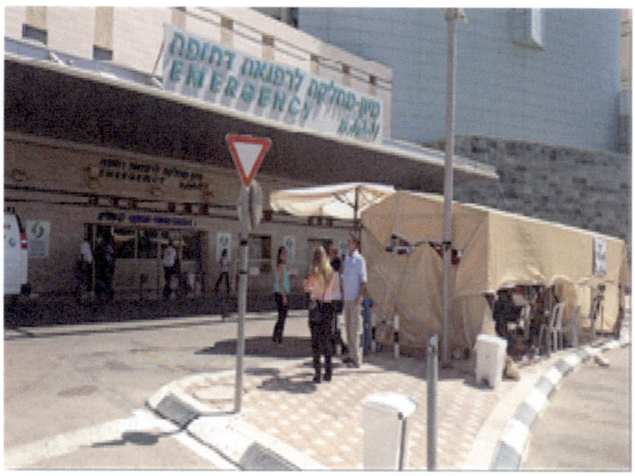

Fig. 6.3 Designated "media tent" at the Soroka hospital in Israel, in front of the entrance to the ER during operation in Gaza 2014 (photo: David Ratner, RHCC)

journalist is not at the scene, curious citizens will "replace" professional journalist and provide amateur video from any event in no time.

Lessons learned from past MCI have led Israeli hospitals to deal with this situation proactively, rather than waiting on regulations and laws to be passed.

In recent years, hospitals have "established" designated journalist areas near the emergency rooms, where ambulances arrive, or near helicopter landing pads. Journalists are permitted to report activity from these areas only. For example, in 2014, during Operation Protective Edge, Soroka Hospital set up a special tent for reporters. The same proactive approach happened at the "Barzilay" hospital in the city of Ashkelon that was bombed by rockets from the Gaza strip (Fig. 6.3).

Hospital administrators have started to assist journalists in such designated areas, by setting up tents and providing food, drinks, chairs, fans, electricity, Wi-Fi, etc., for the journalists. Along with that, the hospitals now clarify to journalists that these are the designated areas for all news coverage, and clearly specify off limit areas such as operating rooms, shock-trauma rooms, etc.

Israeli hospitals, via hospital spokespersons, are now using the same tool that journalists use to transmit real-time information in real time: instant messaging applications (in Israel, one of the most intensively used such applications is "WhatsApp," but any other type of instant messaging application that allows transmission of text, pictures, or video clips works). The experience of spokespersons in Israeli hospitals has shown that a widespread and informed dissemination of information can neutralize the fear (by journalists) that "the hospital is trying to hide something" or that media competitors are "receiving better or different information."

The Israeli experience shows that this approach is also suitable for journalists: they enjoy reasonable working conditions and constant updates from doctors and staff members.

From this point of view, the Israeli experience led to a WIN–WIN situation.

References

1. Schenk E, Wijetunge G, Mann NC, Lerner EB, Longthorne A, Dawson D. Epidemiology of mass casualty incidents in the United States. Prehosp Emerg Care. 2014;18(3):408–16.
2. International Federation of Red Cross and Red Crescent Societies-IFRC. World Disasters Report Resilience: saving lives today, investing for tomorrow: 2016. http://www.ifrc.org/Global/Documents/Secretariat/201610/WDR%202016-FINAL_web.pdf. Accessed 23 July.
3. Landwehr PM, Carley KM. Social media in disaster relief. In: Data mining and knowledge discovery for big data. Berlin Heidelberg: Springer. p. 225–57.
4. Smith SM, Gorski J, Vennelakanti HC. Int J Emerg Manag. 2010;7(3–4):209–20.
5. Lahad M. BASIC Ph: the story of coping resources. Commun Stress Prev. 1997;1:117–45.
6. American Psychiatric Association. Diagnostic and statistical manual of mental disorders. 5th ed. Washington, DC: Author; 2013.
7. Hirshberg A, Holcomb JB, Mattox KL. Hospital trauma care in multiple-casualty incidents: a critical view. Ann Emerg Med. 2001;37(6):647–52.
8. Mehta S. Disaster and mass casualty management in a hospital: how well are we prepared? J Postgrad Med. 2006;52(2):89.
9. Qureshi K, Gershon RR, Sherman MF, Straub T, Gebbie E, McCollum M, Erwin MJ, Morse SS. Health care workers' ability and willingness to report to duty during catastrophic disasters. J Urban Health. 2005;82(3):378–88.
10. Figley CR. Traumatic stress: the role of the family and social support system. In: Figley CR, editor. Trauma and its wake. Vol. II. Traumatic stress theory, research, and intervention. New York: Brunner/Mazel; 1986. p. 39–54.
11. Bride BE. The impact of providing psychosocial services to traumatized populations. Stress Trauma Crisis. 2004;1:29–46.
12. Badger K, Royse D, Craig C. Hospital social workers and indirect trauma exposure: an exploratory study of contributing factors. Health Soc Work. 2008;33(1):63–71.
13. Gagin R, Cohen M, Peled-Avram M. Family support and victim identification in mass casualty terrorist attacks: an integrative approach. Int J Emerg Ment Health. 2005;7(2):125–31.
14. Flannery RB, Everly GS. Crisis intervention: a review. Int J Emerg Ment Health. 2000;2(2):119–26.
15. Mason KE, Urbansky H, Crocker L, Connor M, Anderson MR, Kissoon N, Task Force for Pediatric Emergency Mass Critical Care. Pediatric emergency mass critical care: focus on family-centered care. Pediatr Crit Care Med. 2011;12(6):S157–62.
16. Walsh F. Strengthening family resilience. New York: Guilford Publications; 2015.

17. Shaw JM, Young JM, Butow PN, Badgery-Parker T, Durcinoska I, Harrison JD, Davidson PM, Martin D, Sandroussi C, Hollands M, Joseph D. Improving psychosocial outcomes for caregivers of people with poor prognosis gastrointestinal cancers: a randomized controlled trial (Family Connect). Support Care Cancer. 2016;24(2):585–95.
18. Wen JC, Tsai CC, Chen MH, Chang WT. Operation of emergency operating centers during mass casualty incidents in Taiwan: a disaster management perspective. Disaster Med Public Health Prep. 2014;8(5):426–31.
19. Dudas V, Bookwalter T, Kerr KM, Pantilat SZ. The impact of follow-up telephone calls to patients after hospitalization. Am J Med. 2001;111(9):26–30.
20. Gagin R, Unger-Arnov Y, Shinan-Altman S, Tessler A. The suffering is similar—is the treatment equal? An intervention with Arab terror injured. Soc Work Health Care. 2011;50(5):376–89.
21. Figley CR. Compassion fatigue: psychotherapists' chronic lack of self care. J Clin Psychol. 2002;58(11):1433–41.
22. Miller M. Working in the midst of unfolding trauma and traumatic loss: training as a collective process of support. Psychoanal Soc Work. 2003;10(1):7–25.
23. Nossek H, Limor Y. The Israeli paradox: the military censorship as a protector of the freedom of the press. Research in social problems & public policy. Vol. 19. Emerald Group Publishing Ltd; 2011.
24. Poushter J. Smartphone ownership and internet usage continues to climb in emerging economies. Pew Research Center; Feb 2016.

Nurses and Nursing in Mass Casualties Incidents

7

Ben Rozenblit

Before we begin our desiccation of the unique contribution and role of nurses in MCI, its best to first understand the phenomenon itself.

Intuitively and historically, the definition of an MCI was influenced by the absolute number of injured in the event. However, today, the more correct definition is:

> An event that ***overwhelm*** the local healthcare system, with a number of casualties that vastly *exceeds* the **local** *resources* and capabilities in a **short period** of *time* [1].

Such an event is possible by: natural disasters, transportation accidents, industrial accidents, manmade terror attacks, and many more.

From that definition we can learn that such an event is possible in every country/hospital and health care system, and not only that, but it can and will, happen by surprise and in the worst time possible. It is not a question of *if*, but a question of *when and how*.

In order to understand the scope of those incidents, let's look at some numbers and trends: according to the annual disaster statistical review 2016, "the numbers and trends," by the Centre for Research on the Epidemiology of Disasters (CRED) [2], the total number of people affected by disasters in 2016 (569.4 million) was the highest since 2006, far above its 2006–2015 annual average (224.1 million). The estimated economic losses from natural disasters in 2016 (US$ 153.9 billion) was the fourth highest since 2006; almost 12% above the annual 2006–2015 damages average (US$ 137.6 billion).

According to the Institute for Economics and Peace "global terrorism index 2017 [3]," two-thirds of all countries experienced a terrorist attack in 2016.

B. Rozenblit (✉)
RN, MPH. Emergency and Disaster Management, Tel Aviv University, Tel Aviv, Israel

Emergency Medicine Department, Sheba Medical Center, Ramat Gan, Israel

Nursing School, Tel HaShomer, Ramat Gan, Israel

Y. Kluger et al. (eds.), *WSES Handbook of Mass Casualties Incidents Management*, Hot Topics in Acute Care Surgery and Trauma,
https://doi.org/10.1007/978-3-319-92345-1_7

In 2016, OECD countries experienced the most deaths from terrorism since the September 11 attacks in 2001. There has been a 67% increase in attacks and a nearly 600% increase in deaths from terrorism since 2014. In 2016, the terrorist organization's activities affected 308 cities in 15 countries around the world, four more than the previous year.

Many more data are available in those documents and others like them, but the numbers are clear, and they are reviling a hard reality that all that are dealing with emergency preparedness must deal with: mass casualties, whether they are caused by a flood, hurricane, tornado, earth quake, or mass shooting, are here, and the medical system must be prepared for them as soon as possible.

Mass Casualties Incidents are not a new phenomenon. One would expect from the international health care systems to be prepared for such events, especially in light of the fact that all systems are being/were or will be affected by them at some point in time or another. A paper published in February 2016 in the World Journal of Emergency Surgery by Ben-Ishay et al. wanted to check this preparedness status. The surprising result was: "*the vast unfortunate experience of many countries around the world did not translate into a massive preparedness of hospitals towards a shattering event such as an MCI* [1]".

In other words, although there is a clear necessity to be strongly prepared for those incidents, most of the hospitals/medical systems are not.

To be fully prepared for a MCI, it takes all levels of the countries health care system.

In this chapter, I want to focus on improving the preparedness of the emergency department to a MCI, with the emphasis on the preparations that are being done by nurses.

Before we dive into the preparations themselves, first I would like to take a look at the unique characteristics of nurses and to demonstrate that nurses are one the most important professions in all aspects concerning MCI. The way I decided to do so is by looking at the historical connection between a nurse and emergencies and disasters.

A bit of history—what is so special about nurses and why do we need them in emergencies?

Nurses have been a part of disaster preparedness and response as long as nurses have existed. Although the early nurses who responded to emergencies during historic events have been something other than the fully educated, licensed, professional nurses as we know them today. But still, their described role then is consistent with a lot of the modern understanding of nursing:

attention to the injured or ill individual
assuring provision of water, food, clean dressings, and bedding
providing relief from pain and even something small as offering a human touch that says "I care [4]".

If we look at some specific examples from the history books, we find there are some examples of this historical connection between nurses and emergencies [5].

Pictures from the 1919 influenza epidemic show nurses caring for large numbers of patients placed on cots in rooms more similar to barns than wards.

In the pre-antibiotic era, the major response to any large disease outbreak was comfort and support until the disease ran its course. In the late twentieth century, such was the initial response to what we now know as HIV and AIDS. In cities where this epidemic struck early, large numbers of seriously ill patients were admitted to hospitals for the purpose of receiving good, basic nursing care. This was all that could be done in the absence of any definitive treatment.

Wartime has also added to our understanding of human caring and response to emergencies and disasters. Nurses contributed to this learning, as well as the caring and response.

The origins of nursing, as we know it today, are often traced to the Crimean War experiences of **Florence Nightingale.**

Long histories and many Nightingale biographies are talking about the different methods that she used. The most important one is the presence of disciplined nurses committed to cleanliness and comfort. That in itself allowed more ill and injured soldiers to survive than would otherwise have been the case.

Perhaps even more significant is the later contribution of Miss Nightingale to the decrease in morbidity and mortality of the wounded soldiers through: application of basic statistical analysis, infection control measures, and what we would now consider quality improvement procedures.

Staying in nurses and wars, at the time of the First World War, the hospital units that traveled to Europe were composed of volunteer units, consisting of physicians and nurses from hospitals or communities coming together to fill the essential need for a health presence during and after battle. By World War II, formally organized nursing services had become a part of the military. Nurses in the military often had first exposure to the advances in health care that wartime exigencies stimulated, such as: the use of penicillin, the use of triage, and advanced trauma care [5].

Public health emergencies and nursing:

Nurses have historically played important roles in everyday, local public health emergencies. When a community is challenged by extreme weather, and many families and individuals are isolated, public health nurses work systematically to be sure that no one is abandoned, often traveling with public works crews for access to isolated areas.

As an emergency leads to the establishment of temporary shelters, public health nurses are routinely assigned to assist in triage and screening for health problems, administration of first aid and psychological support, implementation of infection control procedures, and monitoring, so that the congregate living situation does not lead to an outbreak of disease.

To conclude the historical part of this chapter: this part has highlighted some of the historic involvement of nurses in response to emergencies, whether caused by humans or by natural forces.

Without attempting to present an exhaustive listing of activities performed by nurses in emergencies, in past times and in present, the fundamental goal of nursing is to assist individuals to their highest possible level of functioning in the face of health and illness challenges, is never more needed than under emergency conditions.

So, once we emphasized the non-detachable connection between nursing and nurses and emergencies/mass casualties incidents, now I would like to dive back into the specific roles and responsibilities of nurses in preparing their hospital ED for such an event.

However with that being said, one would claim that this type of preparation is almost an impossible task, because every event/health care system/hospital is different. Because of the many differences, there is no only one way of good, professional nursing in an MCI. Nevertheless, there are common professional tasks that nurses take in an MCI, from the emergency department point of view, and those can be summarized as: "Taking care of all the little things and gluing it all together."

This will be my "anchor" and predisposition along this part of the chapter.

So what do nurses do in an MCI? This huge question can be summarized as:

They make sure that everything is prepared **before** the event, taking care of all the "little things" **during** the event (that without them it is impossible to do anything), help to close the event **after** everything is over and finally, they organize the department so it will be ready for the next one.

7.1 Before the Event

"You cannot build a dream on a foundation of sand" said *T.F. Hodge*. Although he was talking about something different, but it is still very true in regards to our subject, and in particular to: a **MCI protocol**.

A pre-made protocol is a must have, because trying to decide what to do in a time of extreme pressure is almost an impossible task. MCI protocols usually exists (if your hospital/health care system is lacking of one, I strongly suggest to write it as soon as possible), and they are the products of the senior management.

But what is the connection between those protocols and nurses? They can, and should, transform them from a huge pile of hard to read pages to an easy and practical tool to use in times of stress.

A small example: the original protocol of the Ministry of Health of Israel is about 83 pages [6], and the protocol of my hospital (Sheba Medical Center) is about 140 pages [7], impossible in a time of stress. In my ED, we prepared a short version of the same protocol, but not only that, we used it in a form a checklist, where each staff member according to the task that he needs to fill gets it in a small folder.

Those folders need to be in a place where they are easy to find, and everyone knows where they are (in the picture below: a folder with a writing: "nurse in charge of wing 2").

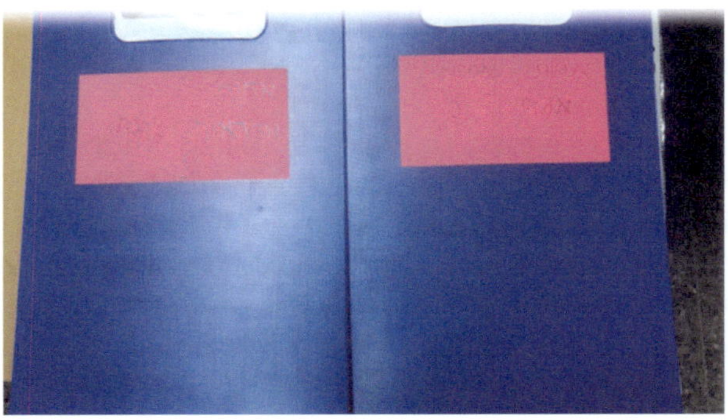

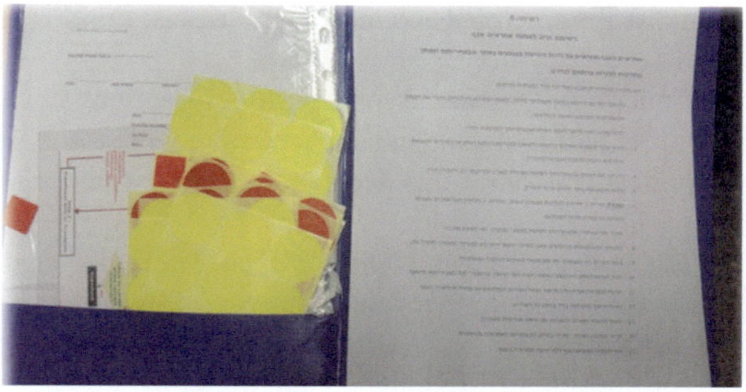

Above is the folder when it is open. Inside there is a specific part of the protocol and a checklist mentioning what there is to do in this site in an alphabetical order.

Managing the man power—**Get more people**—there is no such thing as to many nurses/doctors in a true MCI!

Don't trust your memory, use prepared-in-advance list of essential personal.

A couple of ways to get more people:

1. Public address system (PA system) by the hospital speakers
2. A group call by text/beeper/phone
3. Calling by the "hand-held fan method"—it is a calling method in which one person is calling two more, those two are calling four more, and so on.
4. Calling by a radio or a television

Each hospital calling system and the list itself, needs to be updated three to four times a year and to be tested to see that it works.

Knowing "who's who"—Because there are a lot of staff members at the event, and many are not "organic staff," it is important to know who is who right at the beginning of the event, before "all hell breaks loose."

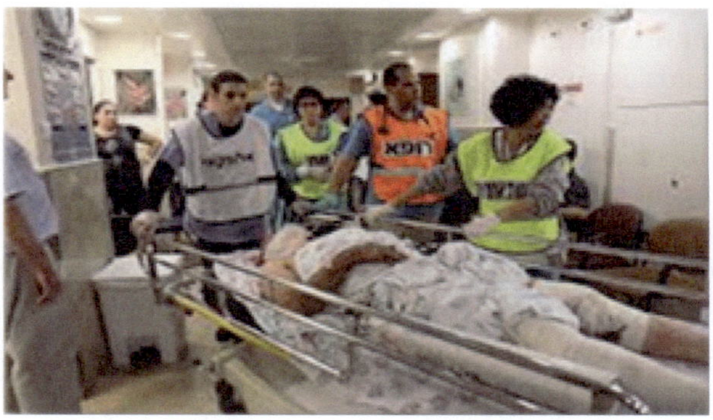

Above there is a picture of medical staff in a time of a MCI. On the left, there is a staff member with a writing of "Hospital attendant." The women with the yellow marking are nurses, and the man with the orange sign is a doctor.

Command and control—this is a huge subject, but from the nurses prospective it can be summarized as: Know in advance who is in charge of what.

The first step in distributing roles and responsibilities is: **making the decision** to declare a MCI.

Because that kind of declaration is one with very serious consequences and financial concerns, it is best to decide in advance how to make and who makes this critical step. It is preferred to leave this decision to the most senior managing position possible.

MCI usually starts in the pre-hospital phase. Once they understand that this is no ordinary event, they are letting the relevant hospital/s know about the event, giving them some time to prepare.

Whether if in your hospital EMS calls are answered by a doctor or whether by nurse, the first step to take is to make sure that the call is not a prank.

If in fact you are facing a MCI, the Head nurse or the nurse in charge, will notify the general manager of the hospital about it, and only he will decide to call the code.

Once the MCI is declared there are key positions that need to be filled.

I will go over on some of them, mainly the ones of nurses.

Head nurse, before the event begins, together with the ED doctor in charge, will do rounds across the ED and divide the existing patients there into three groups: those who need to be hospitalized but, they are waiting for a bed or are in the end of their medical workup but yet with no decision, will go straight to the wards. Those who can be discharged but again, with no such decision, will be discharged at once. The third group (should be the smallest one), those who are at that point can't go anywhere, those will be transferred to the remaining area at the ED and will continue to recieve care in time of the event. Those patients will need specific staff members, who will be in the ED but will not be able to help with the MCI. The purpose of all this re-arrangement: "making room for the incoming injured."

During the event the head nurse will be in charge of the event from the nursing and logistic spectrum. She will usually be right in the center of the ED and in direct communication with other sites managers. She is also assigning the nursing staff to the different work sites.

Trauma Nurse Coordinator—usually during the event will be by the side of the head of the trauma department ("Traumatologist"), helping taking care of the most critically injured patients. After the event has finished, a special team, led by the trauma nurse coordinator will go to all the wards where injured were hospitalized, and help the teams there/make sure, that all are in order and no further help is needed.

Head nurse of the hospital—will notify all staff members relevant to the event and help the ED head nurse in every way the she needs. Will be a part of the hospital Emergency headquarters.

Other than those senior charge nurses, there will be a nurse, alongside the doctor, in charge of every site in the ED. I will discuss about them and their responsibilities, a bit later in the chapter.

Before the MCI reaches your ED, you have to make sure that other very important personal are notified about the event and that they are getting ready. Usually the notification to them goes through the receptionist, but as the charge nurse, you have to make sure/help to get this job done, "the time is on the essence."

Logistic manager—He works very closely with the head nurse and the doctor in charge (under their Giddens). He is responsible for the sanitary workers, drivers, putting signs of the different sites, bringing the equipment carts and makes sure that "other important personal" are present, such as: admin employees, people to "run errands," people who are responsible for oxygen cylinders and more. Another very important job that he has is to be responsible for the **registry team**.

Manager of the blood bank—supposed to come to the ED and be in charge of making sure that the right patient receives the right blood product at the right time. He also manages the blood supply.

Security—are responsible for clearing all the roads leading to the ED and directing essential personal to the right location (keep in mind that closing the roads to cars and clearing them for the ambulances will prevent the medical personal as the other "common people" from getting to the ED. Make sure that they know who needs to be there and who's not). Another job that they have is making sure that at the time of MCI the only people in the ED are those who need to be there, closing the ED so that no family members or press will be allowed to enter.

A quick summary of command and control, as we can see, it is not "a one man show." The command needs to be **decentralized**, but regular updates to the hospital Emergency headquarters are crucial.

The hospital Emergency headquarters—include among others: Hospital manager, Nursing manager, Administration manager, Emergency coordinator, someone from human resources, and more. The biggest role of the headquarters is to supply the best framework to the MCI staff in handling the event.

So, we got the personal and the framework for the event; now we need to organize the ED in a form of different working sites. The main idea is: in order to be able to work in order in a chaos environment you have to "**divide and concur**," meaning divide your ED into different sites so it will be easier to control.

Forward triage—This site is under the responsibility of one of the senior ED doctors and a senior ED nurse. Other staff members who are there—security personal and registry personal. Two major things are happening there: deciding which site the injured needs to be sent to and first aid in a form of stopping bleeding through a tourniquet and helping problems with A/B through "ambu" ventilation.

The Immediate site—those are the most critical patients who have immediate danger to one of their vital systems or an organ. The estimates are that from all the injured about a one third are those.

Key points about the site: One way movement!—x-ray/medical ward/OR. Authorized personal only! Needs special equipment and lots of it. A doctor and a nurse manager.

The "Waiting site"—those are patients with no immediate danger but may require different tests/treatment/hospitalization or discharge. The estimates are that from all the injured about a two thirds are those. Because they can be sent home from this site you got to have a **discharge station/site.**

The purpose of this station/site is to make sure that all got all of their treatment, vaccines if needed (DT/HBV), referral to a clinic, and so on.

The patient will be discharged **only after a 6-h stay at least**.

This site and others like it ("not critical patients") have also other needs such as food and drinks, mental support, information, and more. All of those are under the responsibility of the site nurse through the logistic manager.

Delay before evacuation—In case of inability of the hospital to care for the injured that arrived there (to many victims or lack of a certain profession such as neurosurgery and others), the hospital will become a triage hospital and will transfer the injured to other hospitals. In Israel, the order for that needs to come through the Ministry of Health and will be coordinated with Home Front Command medicine.

Managers of this site are a doctor, nurse, and someone from logistics.

Important to remember about this site: Before the patient can be transferred, the doctor needs to declare certain things such as the way the patient needs to be transferred—either needing supervision of a paramedic/nurse/doctor or special equipment such as a vent, drugs, and also what to notify in advance to the receiving hospital.

Before going, the nurse in charge of this site must make sure that the patient has with him all discharge papers, demographic details of the patient, and a photo of the patient. What was his condition at time of discharge, the name and phone number of the doctor who treated him and what kind of tests (laboratory, X-ray, etc.) did he do and what medicine he got.

Everything will be in two copies, one for each hospital. The information about the transfer will pass to the hospital's Emergency headquarters as well as to public information center.

Dying/critically injured—In case of a large event, those patients will receive a low priority.

Very important to remember: direction to this site is only after an evaluation in the ED and not directly from the triage area! It needs to be separate from the main area.

Primary goal is to ease the pain. In case of casualties, the rule is to leave the police to deal with photographs, ID, registry, etc.

Traumatic stress victims—a victim of this sort will be declared as such only after a primary checkup with the doctor, usually the doctor at the "waiting site."

This site needs to be away from all the other sites, preferably in a quiet remote location. Main staff members here are social workers, psychologists, and mental health personnel.

A basic algorithm to suggest number and layout of the different medical personnel:

Blood bank manager	Social worker	Sanitar/ driver	Nurses assistant	Registry	Nurse	Doctor	Profession/ severity of injury
1 for all sites	–	1:3	1:5	1:2	1:1	1:1	Immediate
	1:20	1:10	1:10	1:5	1:5	1:10	Waiting
–	1:5	1:20	1:10	1:20	1:10	1:5 Psychiatrist	Stress reaction

After re-arranging your ED, getting the right people there, and taking care of the framework for the event, and right before the first victim has arrived… you need **more equipment!**

Equipment—(if we are discussing nurses, it is a known fact, even if it is an informal one, that nurses taking care of equipment).

Because this is another huge subject I will give only key points about it:

The equipment must be arranged in carts (pre-made), where on every cart must be a sign for what it is used for (to which site it needs to go to and a check list of what is in there). Every now and then, all equipment must be checked to make sure that it is ready when needed.

Every staff member needs to know where the carts are placed, so even if the MCI will happen in the middle of the night, where usually the more junior staff is present, they will all know how to begin the preparations until more senior staff arrives. The responsibility of deploying the carts is on the logistic manager under the giddens of the charge nurse.

Some of the special carts are:

1. A and B cart—a breathing cart. Filled with "ambu" devices, laryngoscopes, ET tubs, and so on. Will be deployed at the forward triage site and the immediate site.
2. Children's cart
3. Burn victim's cart—filled with sterile sheets, bottles of saline, ointments such as "silverol," and more.
4. Orthopedic cart—filled with splinting devises, equipment for sowing wounds, ointments such as "polydine," casts, and more.
5. Carts for unconventional MCIs such as biological MCI and chemical MCI

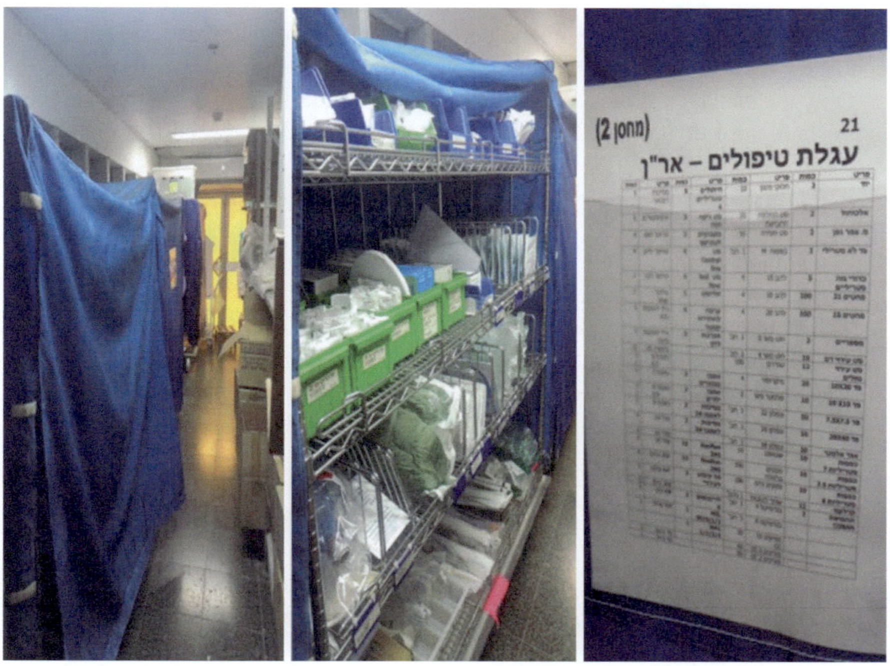

Above, we can see an example from "Sheba Hospital" This is one of the site's carts. On the right, we see a check list of what is in the cart. Below, the middle picture, we see a sign in red saying where this cart needs to go.

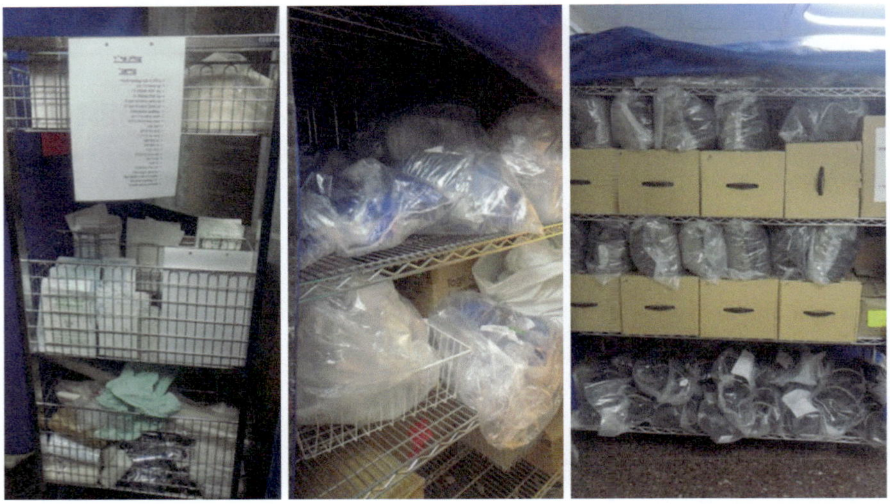

Above are more examples of carts. On the left is the triage cart. In the middle the A and B cart and on the right is an unconventional MCI cart.

7.2 End of the Mass Casualties Incident

It is important not only to begin and continue the MCI in a correct way, but also to end it.

Only the manager of the MCI—The Head of Trauma—will declare that the event is finished, until then, the ED will continue to work in the "special form" that was discussed.

After this declaration was made, a couple of major things need to happen:

1. A team led by the trauma nurse will go and assist the different wards where the injured were hospitalized in every way that is needed.
2. The head nurse of the ED, together with the rest of the nursing staff, will return the ED to his original state before the event.
3. One of the senior ED nurses will take all the MCI carts and equipment, and together with other non-medical personal will fill in the missing equipment and return them back to storage.
4. A senior doctor together with a nurse, will go to the remaining area of the ED where the "third group of patients" remained, and assist them in whatever way is needed.
5. The Head nurse, together with the head of the ED and other essential personal, will meet in the hospital's headquarters to summarize the event.
6. "Back to reality."

To summarize this chapter, I would like to leave you with a very important but easy to remember tip: **KISS**—keep it simple, stupid, meaning—a MCI is not an event in which you trust your memory or trying to "reinvent the wheel."

This is an event in which everything should run automatically. With that said, be prepared in advance **but** expect surprises. One last thing, don't trust technology! In the worst time possible it will fail you. Use manual charts, simple equipment, not very sophisticated vents. Use the simplest communication methods—"runners" or megaphones.

> Everything should be made as simple as possible, but not simplier.
> *Albert Einstein*

References

1. Ben-Ishay O, et al. Mass casualties incidents: time to engage. World J Emerg Surg. 2016;11:8.
2. Centre for Research on the Epidemiology of Disasters (CRED) Institute of Health and Society (IRSS). The numbers and trends. Université catholique de Louvain—Brussels, Belgium. Annual disaster statistical review 2016.
3. Measuring and understanding the impact of terrorism. Institute for Economics and Peace. Global Terrorism Index. 2017.
4. The contribution of nursing and midwifery in emergencies. Report of a WHO Consultation. Geneva: WHO Headquarters; 22–24 Nov 2006.
5. The role of the nurse in emergency preparedness. J Obstet Neonatal Nurs. 2012;41(2):322–24.
6. State of Israel, Ministry of Health, MCI protocol. July 2011.
7. Haim Sheba Medical Center. Emergency Department. MCI protocol.

Auxiliary Clinical Diagnostics

8

Miklosh Bala and Fausto Catena

In disasters and conventional mass casualty incidents (MCI), a large number of trauma patients need to be screened for traumatic injuries and treated within a relatively short time span in restricted resource circumstances. Guidelines and protocols have been developed to enhance decision-making and stabilization of patients without wasting time on less critical injuries [1].

Diagnostic pathways and treatment in the case of disasters and MCIs are highly dependent on the capacity of the emergency department and the auxiliary services: laboratory facilities, department of radiology, and blood banks. Hospitals in the countries with established trauma system are designated as trauma care "level," ranging from I to III, related to available capacity and resources. Level I hospitals provide the full range of diagnostic, resuscitative, and definitive trauma options [2].

This chapter is focused on auxiliary diagnostics in management of MCI: principles, organization, and surge capacity.

Mass casualty incidents (MCIs) have traditionally been managed according to military protocols. First, the closest receiving hospital is quickly flooded by the number of casualties and can't function as a definitive-care hospital. Second, because more casualties are expected, military protocols allow limiting care to critically injured patients, as they will not survive. It is expected to saturate the unit's ability to treat salvageable victims. Thus, military practice that states that "conventional standards of medical care cannot be delivered to all casualties" was incorporated into civilian systems for managing MCIs [3].

M. Bala (✉)
Trauma and Acute Care Surgery Unit, Hadassah—Hebrew University Medical Center, Jerusalem, Israel
e-mail: rbalam@hadassah.org.il

F. Catena
Emergency Surgery Department, Parma University Hospital, Parma, OH, USA

Y. Kluger et al. (eds.), *WSES Handbook of Mass Casualties Incidents Management*, Hot Topics in Acute Care Surgery and Trauma,
https://doi.org/10.1007/978-3-319-92345-1_8

Civilian and military protocols differ significantly. Civilian protocols are mostly based on inner city scenarios, where transportation times are short and the number of casualties is limited. They are based on "scoop-and-run" when minimal care is given by the prehospital teams [4]. Medical centers are well trained and equipped to manage a limited number of civilian casualties. Transfer of patients to more advanced trauma care will depend on the need for specialized surgical and intensive care capabilities.

The extreme opposite is true for disasters: the number of victims is overwhelming, resources become inadequate, and the level of care is compromised [5].

8.1 Scope of Injuries

8.1.1 Blast Injuries

The injuries inflicted by explosive devices are the result of what has been termed a "multidimensional injury" because four separate mechanisms may play a role [6]. The primary blast effect is caused by the high-speed chemical decomposition of explosive materials [7]. Injuries resulting directly from exposure to the blast are referred to as primary blast injuries and affect gas-containing organs such as the lungs, middle ear, and gastrointestinal tract [8].

Secondary blast injuries occur when blast bomb packed with fragments (Fig. 8.1) and other foreign material at the site of the explosion such as glass and stones strike a potential victim, causing penetrating injuries.

Tertiary blast injuries are the result of the generation of "blast winds," which may cause a victim to be thrown from the blast and then hit against the ground or a rigid object, resulting in blunt force trauma. Burn injuries are caused either by flash burns (hot gases released by the explosion) or by ignition of clothing. Although victims usually sustain a combination of these injuries, it is estimated that 47–57% of severe injuries in survivors and 86% of fatal injuries are the result of the effects of the primary blast [8]. Most of the injuries seen in the Israeli experience after an explosion have been related to secondary and tertiary mechanisms [9].

8.1.2 Gunshot Wounds

The effects of GSW are similar to those seen after military or civilian gunshot incidents. In the Israeli experience, when compared with the injuries incurred after explosions, GSW victims experienced a high proportion of open wounds (63 vs. 53%) and fractures (42 vs.31%) [10].

Victims of blast-induced injuries had a higher incidence of both minor (victims at a distance from the explosion) and critical and fatal injuries (victims in close proximity to the explosion), and were more likely to have multiple body regions involved than after GSW.

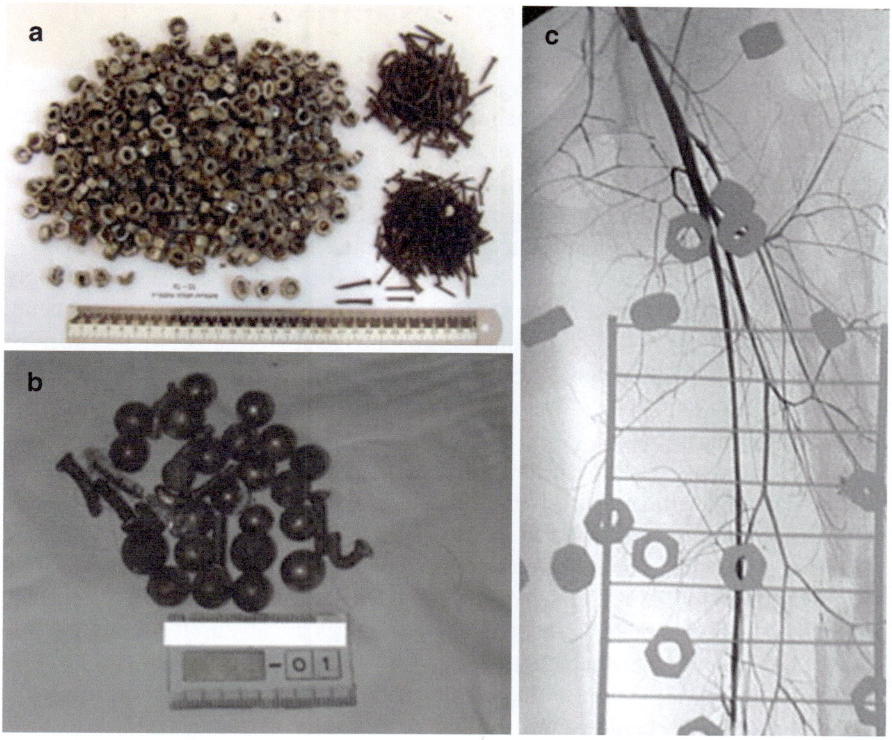

Fig. 8.1 To increase the potential to inflict such injuries, metal particles such as steel pellets, nails, screws, and nuts have been embedded in bombs (**a**, **b**). Bolts seen in the soft tissue of the left thigh during diagnistic angiography of the left femoral artery (**c**)

8.1.3 Other Conventional Mechanism of Injuries

A new type of terrorist attack, the lone terrorist attacker, has become more frequent recently and includes intentional vehicular assaults (IVA) and stabbing attacks [11, 12]. This "lone wolf" phenomenon is characterized by radicals who embark on individual terrorist missions with little or no logistical support [13]. In general, these terrorists have not been operatives of any established terrorist organization, and the current wave of terrorism has not been directed by any organization. To date, these attacks have occurred mostly in the Middle East, Europe, and USA. In Israel, most attacks have centered on the greater Jerusalem area, mainly due to ease of access to Palestinian vehicles. The median number of casualties who were admitted to the ED following an IVA was relatively small (range of 1–5 victims/attack) when compared with the number of casualties following other types of terror acts such as suicide bombing attacks. However, in European experience (Jerusalem, Nice, Berlin) IVA resulted in multiple casualties and can be defined as multiple casualty incidents (MCI, defined as ≥10 casualties arriving at hospital).

8.2 Laboratory Services

Judicious use of the laboratory is essential for accurate diagnosis in the mass-casualty situation. The general management plan is not to overwhelm the laboratory with screening and cut down on laboratory tests of little clinical benefit.

Casualties must continually be moved in a unidirectional flow from ED to other facilities (i.e., ICU, operating room, other hospitals), minimizing or eliminating any use of diagnostic laboratory and imaging tests, while casualty influx continues.

Following in-hospital triage, severely injured patients are assessed accordingly to ATLS protocol and initial lab tests are done. Identification of patients is crucial, and these ID numbers should be maintained unchanged to the end of MCI. The most important lab study is the type and crossmatch, which often can be completed within 20 min of receipt of the blood sample. The recognized risk of "wrong blood in tube" during MCI is high [14].

Arterial blood gases are also useful in the initial assessment period especially in patients exposed to primary blast. Arterial blood gases are repeated at least every 6 h and more frequently in severely injured patients [15]. Baseline labs collected in bleeding patients to guide resuscitation (complete blood count, biochemistry panel and coagulation profile). But for most trauma patients, serum electrolytes, coagulation parameters, cell blood counts, and other common laboratory studies are less useful during the first hours of MCI management in order to decrease a workload of lab services.

If the explosion occurred in an enclosed space or was accompanied by fire, carboxyhemoglobin (HbCO) should be tested. Pulse oximetry readings may be misleading in cases of CO poisoning. Exposure to cyanide (CN), a product of incomplete combustion of plastics, is difficult to measure directly. CN exposure often accompanies CO poisoning. Consider CN poisoning in patients exposed to combustion in an enclosed space (bus, for example) who have an anion gap metabolic acidosis. Treatment for CN poisoning should be started for significantly ill patients while awaiting confirmatory test results. Sodium thiosulfate or hydroxocobalamin are safe and appropriate empiric therapies.

If significant crush injury, compartment syndrome, or severe burns have occurred, emergency physicians should be attentive to the possibility of rhabdomyolysis with resulting hyperkalemia.

As would be expected when entering a mass-casualty scenario, the volume of specimens received in the laboratory rapidly approached maximum capacity. With Israeli experience, the only ones that need initially any lab tests in an MCI situations, are the REALLY, REALLY sick ones (25% or 4 patients in each event) [16]. All the others can wait till the chaos subsides. Those who DO need blood tests, are not different from the "Regular," "Every Day" major trauma patient: blood type and crossmatch and ABG preferably with lactate level. All the rest of the tests that we take are "excess baggage," and are just for "documentation" and "Baseline." The sicker the patient, the less tests are important since the numbers in the OR will be very different after initial resuscitation. However, if the patient is not sick, again, they are not important. Victims triaged to category green (or walking wounded) should not undergo any imaging.

Lab personnel are trained to alert the treating team (often medical director) when there is a shortage of recourses and abnormal results are found for specific patient (hyperkalemia, excessive lactate level, and very low hemoglobin).

8.2.1 Radiology Department in MCI

Imaging examinations during MCI including ultrasound, radiography (XR), CT, and angiography can be used to improve the accuracy of triage in MCIs. Imaging utilization has been reported as high as 93% of victims in one study in the military setting of three explosive MCIs in Iraq in 2008 [17].

Radiologic images can help determine which patients will be triaged to immediate surgery and which will be followed up conservatively, often with use of repeated radiologic examination. Large numbers of casualties whose complicated injuries are due to blast and shrapnel require the most sophisticated imaging but are often admitted with no or minimal early warning to the ED during a brief period [18]. Early activation of MCI hospital protocol should include radiology department. Personnel who must be notified are the department chair, chief technician, and radiologist and radiologic technicians on call [19]. Additional personnel, including potentially any and all radiologists, radiographers, and administrative staff, should be recruited on the basis of the size of the MCI.

Radiology department used to be a limited resource and additionally may cause "bottleneck" during MCI. Surge capacity refers to the ability to evaluate and care for an increased volume of patients that challenges or exceeds normal operating capacity [20].

Surge capacity for radiology should include the number of examinations that can be performed simultaneously or in a given time period. Evaluation should include time needed for image transfer, time for image reading and reporting, time for patients to be transferred to and from radiology areas, the capacity of patient waiting areas. Some studies are operator dependent and could be underestimated, if no drills were conducted before real MCI happens.

Before casualties are transported to radiology department facilities, they must undergo assessment by a triage team and the priority is driven by MCI medical director. This is an absolute key point in maintaining control of resources for more urgent patients [21].Victims triaged to category green (or walking wounded) should not undergo any imaging as long as more urgent patients are expected to arrive in the radiology department. Patients tagged "yellow" or urgent typically need at least some basic imaging (chest X-ray or/and US) to detect if they are undertriaged or overtriaged. In patients tagged "red" or critically injured, imaging should be limited if they need to be transferred quickly to the OR (pericardial effusion, large hemothorax, etc.).

If the patient is stable enough, whole-body CT may be performed to detect all possible injuries with high accuracy.

8.2.2 Blood Bank

Blood services worldwide must be prepared to meet demand for blood components needed by casualties of domestic disasters and acts of terrorism. Israel's National Blood Services, operated by Magen David Adom, has extensive experience in managing blood collections and supply in emergencies.

Exsanguinating hemorrhage is a major cause of death in civilian and military casualties. In the US, 10–15% of all RBC units are used to treat injured patients [22].

Surgical studies define 10 units of packed red blood cells (PRBC) as a massive transfusion in patients with severe injury and much recent research has been aimed at them [23, 24].

Trauma centers have evolved massive transfusion protocols that include activation of additional personnel, employment of rapid infusion systems, automatic thawing of plasma, and changes in crossmatching policy. Recent analysis of combat events from Iraq and Afghanistan demonstrates that approximately 20% of casualties will require blood transfusion and 7% will require massive transfusion [25, 26].

Few articles have been written, however, directly addressing the management and resource utilization in mass casualty incidents (MCI). Soffer et al. analyzed 18 consecutive terrorist attacks and found that the number of PRBC units transfused per patient was related to incident size, with smaller incidents (<25 evacuated casualties) having a number of PRBC transfused to patient per incident (PPI) of 0.7 and larger incidents having a PPI of 1.5. Half of the units of PRBCs were required in the first 2 h after the incident [27].

Meticulous monitoring of the both local and national blood inventory is performed daily, and the report is submitted to the governing bodies [28].

The Hadassah BB protocol and contingency plans were created for the management of blood requirements following MCI [29]. The protocol defines certain activation steps which are necessary to ensure adequate blood supply to the Emergency Department (ED), trauma unit, operating room, and Intensive Care Units. Notification of hospital and BB can be performed in several ways. Information regarding an MCI can reach the blood bank either directly from hospital administration, central MDA command, or as has happened on several occasions, through the media and internet. Once the BB has been alerted, it is the responsibility of the BB representative to evaluate/verify the severity of the event, i.e., the number of wounded, attack setting, and expected time of arrival. Recruitment of Central Blood Storage assistance will depend on these factors. Three units of blood expected to prepare for each severe injured and two for mildly injured casualty. Uncrossmached type O- (2 units) delivered to trauma unit. Ten type-A and O PRBC are thawed, as are 10 units of fresh frozen plasma (FFP). Additional BB personnel are recruited. A BB representative arrives in the ED and trauma unit in order to coordinate blood transfusion and ensure proper handling of blood samples. Priority is given to discharge type-specific blood over type O.

An average of 66.8 PRBCs (PPI = 4.02) was transfused during the 5 attacks with 10 or more admitted victims while the average for the remaining 12 attacks was

15.8 PRBC/attack (PPI = 3.8). However, there was much variability and in 2 attacks 36 and 56 PRBCs were transfused when only 6 and 3 patients, respectively, were admitted from the ER.

Preparing blood for many victims following an MCI can challenge any blood bank. Massive transfusions pose an even greater challenge. Our data show that up to 10% of patients will require 10 or more PRBCs within the initial 24 h of admission. This is similar to data from Iraq (8%), where most of casualties were injured by a combination of blast and penetrating injury [30–32]. But again, it was much higher than previously reported from Israel (4.7%) [27].

In London bombing attack, 264 units of blood products were used in the first 15 h of the major incident including a total of 130 units of packed red blood cells, 46 units of fresh frozen plasma, 70 units of cryoprecipitate, and 11 pools of platelets.

Hematology staff were diverted from other areas to support the usual two transfusion technicians and all non-urgent requests for blood crossmatching and typing were postponed [33].

The most frequently reported adverse event associated with blood transfusion is the administration of the wrong type of blood to the patient, which can, at worst, result in a fatal hemolytic reaction. The risk of error is particularly high in an emergency situation, when several patients are admitted concomitantly and some are unidentified. To make this process safer, barcode systems have been developed. However, the use of these devices is not always eliminating mistakes in an emergency.

It is the responsibility of the BB representative to evaluate/verify the severity of the event and report to BB director and EMS services about current storage and especially shortage of blood products. The blood bank representative in the ED double checks correct labeling of blood sample tubes and blood request forms as well as the use of 2 ID numbers for each patient prevented errors associated with the management of the wounded in mass casualty events during the first hour after admission [34].

Penetrating injury and multiple body area involved were found in all patient required massive transfusions. Most blood products were given in the first 24 h and particularly in the first 2 h of admission. But uncrossmatched O-PRBC were given to the limited number of casualties in extreme. Initiation of mass casualty event blood bank protocol is utmost important.

Importantly, we stated that transfusion medicine physicians became integral members of the treating team in situations of MCI to promote a rational and safe use of blood products for the management of severely wounded patients.

References

1. American College of Surgeons Committee on Trauma. Advanced trauma life support for doctors: student course manual. 8th ed. Chicago: American College of Surgeons; 2008.
2. Department of Health, Welfare and Sport. Beleidsvisie traumazorg 2006–2010. 2006. http://www.rijksoverheid.nl/bestanden/documenten-en-publicaties/kamerstukken/2006/04/19/beleidsvisietraumazorg-2006-2010/cz-2671397b.pdf. Accessed 6 Sept 2017.

3. Sorting of casualties. In: Bowen TE, Bellamy RF, editors. Emergency war surgery. Washington, DC: US GovernmentPrinting Office; 1988. p. 181–92.
4. Border JR, Lewis FR, Aprahamian C, Haller JA, Jacobs LM, Luterman A. Panel: prehospital trauma care—stabilize or scoop and run. J Trauma. 1983;23:708–11.
5. Frykberg ER. Medical management of disasters and mass casualties from terrorist bombings: how can we cope? J Trauma. 2002;53:201–12.
6. Kluger Y. Bomb explosions in acts of terrorism—detonation, wound ballistics, triage and medical concerns. Isr Med Assoc J. 2003;5:235–40.
7. Wightman JH, Gladish SL. Explosions and blast injuries. Ann Emerg Med. 2001;37:664–78.
8. Mayorga MA. The pathology of primary blast overpressure injury. Toxicology. 1997;121:17–28.
9. Peleg K, Aharonson-Daniel L, Stein M, et al. Gunshot and explosion injuries: characteristics, outcomes and implications for care of terror related injuries in Israel. Ann Surg. 2004;239(3):311–8.
10. Aharonson-Daniel L, Klein Y, Peleg K, ITG. Suicide bombers form a new injury profile. Ann Surg. 2006;244(6):1018–23.
11. Almogy G, Kedar A, Bala M. When a vehicle becomes a weapon: intentional vehicular assaults in Israel. Scand J Trauma Resusc Emerg Med. 2016;24(1):149.
12. Rozenfeld M, Givon A, Peleg K. Violence-related versus terror-related stabbings: significant differences in injury characteristics. Ann Surg. 2018;267(5):965–70. https://doi.org/10.1097/SLA.0000000000002143.
13. Reid MJ, Yakeley J. The violent true believer as a "lone wolf"—psychoanalytic perspectives on terrorism. Behav Sci Law. 2014;32:347–65.
14. Milkins C, Berryman J, Cantwell C, Elliott C, Haggas R, Jones J, Rowley M, Williams M, Win N. British Committee for Standards in Haematology Guidelines for pre-transfusion compatibility procedures in blood transfusion laboratories. Transfus Med. 2013;23:3–35.
15. Pizov R, Oppenheim-Eden A, Matot I, Weiss YG, Eidelman LA Rivkind AI, Sprung CL. Blast lung injury from an explosion on a civilian bus. Chest. 1999;115(1):165–72.
16. Aschkenasy-Steuer G, Shamir M, Rivkind A, Mosheiff R, Shushan Y, Rosenthal G, Mintz Y, Weissman C, Sprung CL, Weiss YG. Clinical review: the Israeli experience: conventional terrorism and critical care. Crit Care. 2005;5(9):490–9.
17. Raja AS, Propper BW, Vandenberg SL, Matchette MW, Rasmussen TE, Johannigman JA, et al. Imaging utilization during explosive multiple casualty incidents. J Trauma. 2010;68:1421–4.
18. Almogy G, Rivkind AI. Suicide bombing: the general surgeon's view. In: Shemer J, Shoenfeld Y, editors. Terror and medicine: medical aspects of biological chemical and radiological terrorism. Lengerich: Pabst Science; 2003. p. 409–19.
19. Sosna J, Sella T, Shaham D, Shapira SC, Rivkind A, Bloom AI, Libson E. Facing the new threats of terrorism: radiologists' perspectives based on experience in Israel. Radiology. 2005;237(1):28–36.
20. Franc JM, Ingrassia PL, Verde M, Colombo D, Della Corte F. A simple graphical method for quantification of disaster management surge capacity using computer simulation and process-control tools. Prehosp Disaster Med. 2015;30:9–15.
21. Vanden Berg SL, Davidson SB. Preparation for mass casualty incidents. Crit Care Nurs Clin North Am. 2015;27:157–66.
22. Hess JR, Hiippala S. Optimizing the use of blood products in trauma care. Crit Care. 2005;9:S10–4.
23. Como JJ, Dutton RP, Scalea TM, Edelman BB, Hess JR. Blood transfusion rates in the care of acute trauma. Transfusion. 2004;44:809–13.
24. Johansson PI, Hansen MB, Sorensen H. Transfusion practice in massively bleeding patients: time for a change? Vox Sang. 2005;89:92–6.
25. Beekley AC, Martin MJ, Spinella PC, Telian SP, Holcomb JB. Predicting resource needs for multiple and mass casualty events in combat: lessons learned from combat support hospital experience in operation Iraqi freedom. J Trauma. 2009;66:S129–37.
26. Beekley AC, Starnes BW, Sebesta JA. Lessons learned from modern military surgery. Surg Clin North Am. 2007;87:157–84.

27. Soffer D, Klausner J, Bar-Zohar D, Szold O, Schulman CI, Halpern P, Shimonov A, Hareuveni M, Ben-Tal O. Usage of blood products in multiple-casualty incidents: the experience of a level I trauma center in Israel. Arch Surg. 2008;143:983–9.
28. Shinar E, Yahalom V, Silverman BG. Meeting blood requirements following terrorist attacks: the Israeli experience. Curr Opin Hematol. 2006 Nov;13(6):452–6.
29. Bala M, Kaufman T, Keidar A, Zelig O, Zamir G, Mudhi-Orenshat S, Bdolah-Abram T, Rivkind AI, Almogy G. Defining the need for blood and blood products transfusion following suicide bombing attacks on a civilian population: a level I single-centre experience. Injury. 2015;45:50–5.
30. Propper BW, Rasmussen TE, Davidson SB, Vandenberg SL, Clouse WD, Burkhardt GE, Gifford SM, Johannigman JA. Surgical response to multiple casualty incidents following single explosive events. Ann Surg. 2009;250:311–5.
31. Perkins JG, Cap AP, Spinella PC, Shorr AF, Beekley AC, Grathwohl KW, Rentas FJ, Wade CE, Holcomb JB, 31st Combat Support Hospital Research Group. Comparison of platelet transfusion as fresh whole blood versus apheresis platelets for massively transfused combat trauma patients (CME). Transfusion. 2011;51:242–52.
32. Marshall WB. Resuscitation of combat casualties: unique challenges and lessons learned. AACN Adv Crit Care. 2010;21:279–87.
33. Aylwin CJ, König TC, Brennan NW, Shirley PJ, Davies G, Walsh MS, Brohi K. Reduction in critical mortality in urban mass casualty incidents: analysis of triage, surge, and resource use after the London bombings on July 7, 2005. Lancet. 2006;368(9554):2219–25.
34. Dann EJ, Michaelson M, Barzelay M, Hoffman R, Bonstein L. Transfusion medicine during the summer of 2006: lessons learned in northern Israel. Transfus Med Rev. 2008;22(1):70–6.

Conventional and Interventional Radiology in Mass Casualty Incidents

9

Amos Ofer, Maxim Leiderman, and Nira Beck-Razi

Dealing with MCI has become an increasingly important aspect of modern medicine due to the increase in terrorist and other mass casualty acts. Thus, almost every hospital is expected to be prepared for such incidents [1] which are usually caused by motor vehicle accidents, explosions, shootings, earthquakes, and other naturally caused disasters [2]. Estimates show a continuous rise of terrorist acts: According to the second edition of Global Terrorism Index, there was a five-fold increase in the number of people killed by terrorism from 2000 to 2013, resulting in approximately 18,000 deaths. Some well-known examples of the largest MCIs since 2000 including natural and man-made disasters are: the 9/11 Twin Tower attack (New York, 2001), the Indian Ocean tsunami (2004), the Madrid train bombings (2004), the hurricane Katrina (New Orleans, 2005), the Christchurch earthquake (New Zealand, 2011), the Rana Plaza collapse (Bangladesh, 2013), the Ebola outbreak (West Africa, 2014), the Mina stampede (Mecca 2015), and the Paris terrorist shootings (2015) [1].

The diagnostic radiologist and the interventional radiologist, have a central role in the management of such patients aiming to reduce mortality and morbidity [3]. Every radiologist should be able to recognize the spectrum of injuries inflicted by explosive devices, motor vehicle accidents, and other causes of MCI. Every imaging department including US, CT, and IR units should be trained in managing MCI. In MCI, the medical system is overwhelmed with a temporary disruption of the balance between resources and demands [1–3]. On such occasions, the classic paradigm of medical management of giving optimal treatment to every single patient is shifted

A. Ofer (✉) · M. Leiderman
Department of Medical Imaging, Rambam Health Care Campus, Haifa, Israel
e-mail: a_ofer@rambam.health.gov.il

N. Beck-Razi
Department of Medical Imaging, Rambam Health Care Campus, Haifa, Israel

The Ruth and Bruce Rappaport Faculty of Medicine, Technion-Israel Institute of Technology, Haifa, Israel

Y. Kluger et al. (eds.), *WSES Handbook of Mass Casualties Incidents Management*, Hot Topics in Acute Care Surgery and Trauma,
https://doi.org/10.1007/978-3-319-92345-1_9

towards decreasing mortality and morbidity for the entire population even at the cost of providing potentially less than routine treatment an individual patient [3, 4].

Imaging examinations including ultrasound, radiography (XR), and CT can be used to improve the accuracy of triage in MCIs. Imaging utilization has been reported as high as 93% of victims in one study in the military setting of three explosive MCIs in Iraq in 2008 and 72% of victims in a large civilian airplane crash in 2009 in the Netherlands [1, 5]. In our institute, 79% of physically injured patients admitted during the second Lebanon war underwent imaging in the radiology department [6]. Therefore, imaging providers must be prepared to support treatment teams during activation of MCIs [1].

Thus, the hallmark of MCI is the chaos imposed on the emergency and other event-dependent in-hospital departments. In order to deal with this chaos, the three main issues characterizing MCI involving the radiology department should be addressed:

1. The need for an extensive amount of medical and non-medical personal.
2. Change of the ordinary workflow of the radiology department.
3. Failure of the ordinary cellular phones-based communication.

9.1 Reinforcement of Radiological Staff

One of the main issues in managing MCI is the need for an extensive amount of medical and paramedical personal [3, 4]. Unlike everyday ordinary hospital activities, MCI is characterized by a spike-like burst of activity. Thus, every unit and department needs a predefined set of actions in order to reinforce the personal needed [6]. The best and most practical method is to have a pre-prepared binder in each department containing lists of personal to be called once an MCI has been announced [1]. This binder should also be backed up in the hospital's digital network. Each member of the radiology department should have a pre-planned emergency position which is also listed in the MCI binder. The head of the department, her deputy, and the senior doctor in charge of emergency events are notified immediately by the person receiving the MCI announcement. All directors of paramedical sectors including X-ray technicians, nurses, secretaries, and others are also notified. Upon arriving to the department, each worker is assigned to his/her pre-planned position: teams consisting of X-ray technicians, residents, and senior doctors are sent to the emergency room for US fast examinations. For each CT scanner, a team consisting of at least two radiologists is needed. At least two interventional radiologists are needed in the IR unit and the same for US unit. The most senior radiologist present can reinforce different units on line as needed [7].

9.2 Change of the Ordinary Workflow

Once an MCI has been announced all other non-emergency imaging procedures should be stopped [3, 7] and the patients involved are returned to their wards or discharged from the hospital. Unlike ordinary hospital activities in the setup of

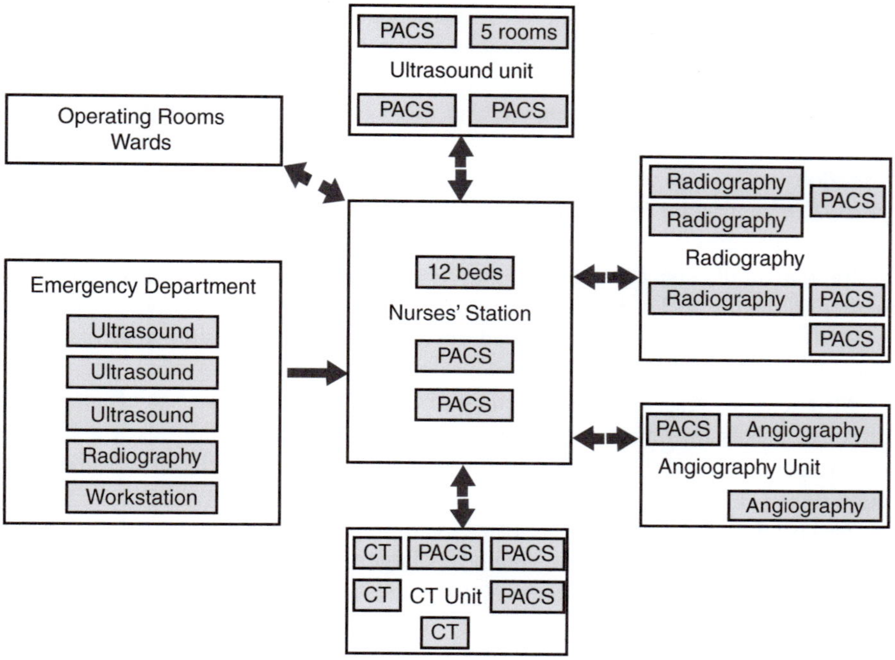

Fig. 9.1 Scheme of the imaging facilities in the radiology and emergency departments during an MCI: Unlike ordinary hospital activities patients are not returned to the emergency room once completing the diagnostic imaging process. This is illustrated by the single direction arrow from the emergency department

MCI, patients are not returned to the emergency room once completing the diagnostic imaging process. Patients should not be returned to the emergency room because of the need to prepare the emergency room for another wave of incoming patients: A pre-planned holding place, reinforced with nurses and clinical doctors, receives these patients before progressing to their next step/station of treatment [6]. This holding place is treated as a temporary extension of the emergency department during the whole MCI period (Fig. 9.1) [6].

Another notable change in the ordinary workflow is the increased usage in US [8]:

9.2.1 FAST in Multiple Casualty Incidents

Effective initial triage, defined as the art of sorting patients according to the severity of their injury, is the key to successfully dealing with a multiple casualty incident (MCI). In order to proceed to further triage and patient management, there is a need for a quick and efficient imaging diagnosing test. FAST [focused abdominal sonography for trauma] can be performed rapidly in the admission area, is repeatable, noninvasive, non-irradiating, and inexpensive. It is widely accepted as an effective initial tool to evaluate trauma victims with suspected blunt abdominal injuries [4, 5, 8, 9].

FAST may play an important role in the work-up of trauma patients in MCI due to the complexity of the injuries. Some controversies remain concerning the role of FAST in penetrating trauma [10]. We believe that FAST has an important part in evaluation of all trauma injuries, whether blunt or penetrating, and should be performed on all of them during the resuscitation phase. Ultrasound is fast, noninvasive, does not involve radiation, portable, and can be integrated into the resuscitation process in the trauma bay without disrupting it.

A negative FAST should be received with caution [4], especially in penetrating abdominal injury, because in such injuries it takes time to develop appreciable hemoperitoneum to be detected by ultrasound. Although the role of FAST in an individual trauma casualty has been reviewed in the literature, a few studies described the role of FAST in MCIs.

Miletic et al. described US screening of mass war casualties as an efficient and effective means for detection and on-site triage of abdominal injuries which were mostly penetrating (90%) with a similar sensitivity and specificity in war and civil conditions [11].

Sarkisian et al. [12] described a successful application of ultrasound after catastrophic earthquake in Armenia, which was largely a crush injury.

In a study we conducted on a 102 soldiers and civilians during the Second Lebanon War, we reported a sensitivity of 75% for hemoperitoneum detection. Injuries encountered were of blunt and penetrating combined. Our results show that FAST as the first imaging examination during continuous arrival phase in a setting of a war conflict-related MCI enabled immediate triage of casualties to laparotomy, CT, or clinical observation.

Due to the moderate sensitivity and the limitation in diagnosing solid organs or hollow viscous injury, a negative FAST in the presence of a strong clinical suspicion must be followed by CT or laparotomy according to clinical judgment [4, 13].

EFAST is known as the Extended FAST and includes examining the pleura for pneumothorax and the pericard for hemopericardium.

The pleura is scanned, to rule out pneumothoraxes when immediate surgery is needed, in order to prevent accumulation of a tension pneumothorax due to positive pressure ventilation in surgery. This can be of a benefit when there is no time or available mobile X-ray machines.

The pericard is examined as a part of the EFAST although its benefit in blunt trauma has been questioned [14].

9.3 Communications

In most modern hospitals, everyday in-house communication is done through personnel held cellular phones. This mode of communication is not sufficient during an MCI because of cellular system overwhelming usage [6]. In order to overcome this limitation, a simple, non-cellular communication system should be prepared. Simple, commercially available, cheap walkie-talkies handheld portable two-way radio transceivers can be used [6]. These should be held by radiological personal stationed in key positions: by the most senior radiological personal stationed in the emergency room, by the director of the department or the senior radiological staff member stationed in the entrance to the radiological department, by the senior radiologist in charge of the CT unit and by the radiologist staff member stationed in the holding place [6]. This will provide a simple and efficient way of maintaining contact between the radiological staff and keeping on line close coordination with the emergency department staff during the whole period of the MCI.

9.3.1 The Role of CT in MCI

CT is the modality of choice in multisystem trauma [5, 15] and can be used as a triage tool during an MCI [1, 5]. The protocols used should be simple and standard. A whole body protocol should be used liberally in order to avoid time-consuming discussions in attempts to limit CT coverage to specific body parts [16]. This will also reduce the need for repeated visits to the CT suite [1] because of a missing scan. Whole body CT produces a large number of images which are best viewed using dedicated workstations capable of doing secondary image reformation and 3D viewing [1, 15].

9.3.2 Blast Injuries

In the last decades, a large portion of MCI are caused by terror. These are usually due to various explosive devices that cause blast injuries. Thus, every radiologist should be familiar with this type of injury. This pattern of injury can be complex, unpredictable, and diagnostically challenging [17]. Characteristically, explosive injuries have a higher proportion of critically injured patients compared to other multitrauma events [17].

9.3.2.1 Blast (Explosive) Injury

Explosive injuries are classified into four categories: Primary, Secondary, Tertiary, and Quaternary [18]. Patients may be affected by one or more injuries from different categories [17, 19].

Primary Injuries

These are a result of the initial very high pressure wave impacting at air–liquid interfaces [15, 17]. The primary high pressure wave spreads radially at the speed of sound generating winds of high velocity up to several hundred km/h [19]. The degree of tissue injury is directly related to the proximity of the victim to the explosion [17]. Several systems and organs are prone to primary blast injury: limbs and earlobes may be traumatically amputated. Rupture of the inner ear, eardrum, blast lung injury, and viscous perforation of the gastrointestinal tract may occur. Primary blast lung injury may lead to an immediate death due to massive cerebral or coronary air embolism (Fig. 9.2) [17].

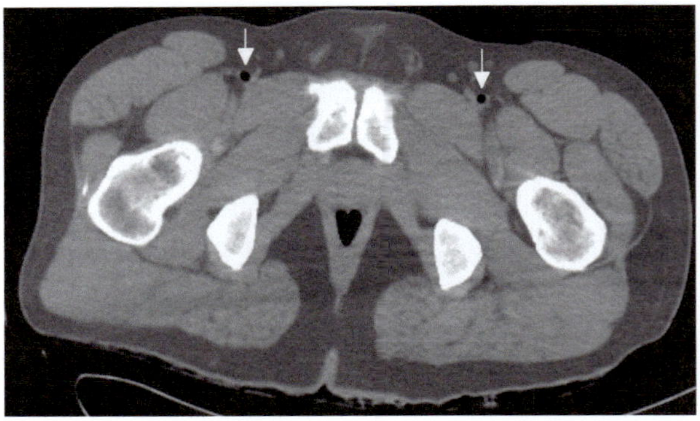

Fig. 9.2 Primary blast injury in a 30-year-old soldier. Air replacing blood is noted in the superficial femoral arteries below the inguinal ligaments (arrows)

Secondary Injuries

These are caused by flying bomb fragments and debris, metallic and nonmetallic, causing penetrating trauma similar to wounds seen in combat trauma [15, 17, 19].

Tertiary Injuries

These occur as a result of a long phase of negative pressure displacing the whole body that impacts onto fixed objects. This may cause blunt and penetrating injuries, head and cervical spine as well as orthopedic injuries [18].

Quaternary Injuries

These include all other injuries mainly burns and smoke inhalation [17–19].

9.3.3 Reporting of Radiological Findings

The radiologists should attempt to perform real-time on-site interpretation and communicate verbally [7, 8, 16] as soon as possible with the physicians and staff who are in charge of the patient. Direct verbal communication is essential to decrease confusion and increase efficiency especially regarding patients who are in critical condition. It is essential to have designated qualified physicians (e.g., surgeons or anesthesiologists) in the CT, US, or angiography suite accompany such patients. They are needed to monitor and treat any change in the patient's condition during the course of imaging studies or procedures. The verbal communication should be followed with an officially written report. Any change in the interpretation of the radiological finding should be in writing and confirmed by the accompanying clinical physician.

9.3.4 Conclusion of MCI

Announcing the end of an MCE is important because the intensity of work required in this situation cannot continue for a long period of time [3]. As soon as possible, all participants need to meet for a debriefing session to draw conclusions and lessons regarding the MCI. This often results in updates of protocols and determination of where gaps exist in workforce, knowledge, and equipment that needs to be changed for better performance in future MCI [3].

9.4 Interventional Radiology in MCI

Interventional radiology has a twofold role during MCI: diagnosing and treating vascular injuries.

9.4.1 Imaging Modalities in Arterial Injury Diagnosis

Different imaging modalities may be considered in the vascular evaluation of the traumatized patient.

9.4.1.1 Doppler Sonography

The advantages of Duplex sonography are well known. It is a noninvasive examination, mostly not painful, and can be done at the patient's bedside in the Emergency Room or in the Operating Theater [20]. In experienced centers, it offers high sensitivity in comparison to the gold standards: digital angiography and surgery [20, 21]. However, Doppler sonography is a time-consuming method and is highly operator dependent [22].

Moreover, this examination is not feasible in open wounds with large soft tissue defects, with surrounding edema, hematoma, and bony fractures [20, 21]. Duplex sonography is also limited by bulky dressings and orthopedic hardware [21]. In addition, Duplex sonography is focused to the suspected region of injury, while unsuspected pathology may be missed. Thus, US Doppler has little role in MCI.

9.4.1.2 Magnetic Resonance Angiography (MRA)

Magnetic resonance angiography is an excellent tool in the demonstration of vascular structures. However, in the setting of acute vascular trauma in most trauma centers, accessibility and monitoring of the critically wounded patient within the magnet is a major problem and not practical [21, 22]. In addition, with penetrating trauma there may be metal pellets that are not compatible with MRI and may result in artifacts [23]. Thus, MRA has no role in MCI.

9.4.1.3 Conventional Angiography (CA)

In the past, the gold standard in the evaluation of vascular injuries has been invasive conventional angiography [24].

Conventional angiography is a costly and time-consuming procedure that requires the presence of a trained and specialized team including an interventional radiologist, a technician, and a nurse. The time required for the team to arrive at the hospital and the duration of the procedure may delay the definitive treatment that might be critical in a state of emergency [20, 21, 25]. This disadvantage is emphasized in MCI due to the inherent shortage of resources. Thus, conventional angiography has a very limited role in vascular diagnosis in MCI.

Conventional angiography remains the tool of choice in diagnosing or excluding vascular injury when other noninvasive modalities, namely CT-angiography, fail to perform.

Conventional angiography has a major role when endovascular treatment is recommended [25].

9.4.1.4 CT-Angiography (CTA)

Imaging of vascular injuries has undergone a dramatic change since the introduction of Multi-Detector Computerized Tomography (MDCT). Improved CT technology, providing rapid acquisition of thin axial slices, led to the development of CT-angiography. Compared with conventional arteriography, CTA shows excellent sensitivity and specificity in diagnosing occlusive disease in the lower extremities and in other parts of the body [20, 24, 25].

Since 1999 CTA has shown excellent results for imaging traumatic arterial injuries [20–22] and is continuously replacing conventional catheter angiography as it is in other non-traumatic vascular evaluation [20, 24, 26, 27]. According to Soto et al., in an early study in 1999 using a single detector helical CT, and evaluating traumatized extremities, the sensitivity and specificity of CTA were 90–100% and 100%, respectively [26].

The same group published one more study several years later. Based on this study which also used a single detector helical CT, CTA had a sensitivity of 95.1% and a specificity of 98.7% in significant blunt and penetrating trauma to large extremity arteries [27].

In 2017, Madhuripan et al. summarized the use of CTA in emergencies of the extremities and concluded that CTA is currently the first-line investigation for this purpose with high specificity and sensitivity [24].

In addition to the high sensitivity and specificity, CTA offers a number of advantages over conventional angiography. It is a noninvasive examination, readily available in most institutions, it is not as time consuming as conventional arteriography, and it is cost-effective. Moreover, in order to carry out a CTA examination there is no need to assemble a specialized team; it allows the presence of monitoring equipment in close proximity to the critically wounded patient and the clinical team can remain at the CT console observing the patient and the evolving examination [20, 21].

Following data acquisition, multiplanar three-dimensional reconstructions can be easily obtained, facilitating the diagnosis and the planning of further management.

However, axial images should always be reviewed carefully because on the 3D images arterial lumen might be obscured by vascular calcifications as well as by foreign bodies and partial thrombosis (Fig. 9.3) [20, 23].

The advantages of CTA, mainly the speed of the acquisition and the accuracy of the CTA scan make it an ideal diagnostic tool for vascular imaging in MCI. Another very important advantage of CTA is the standardization of the diagnostic procedure.

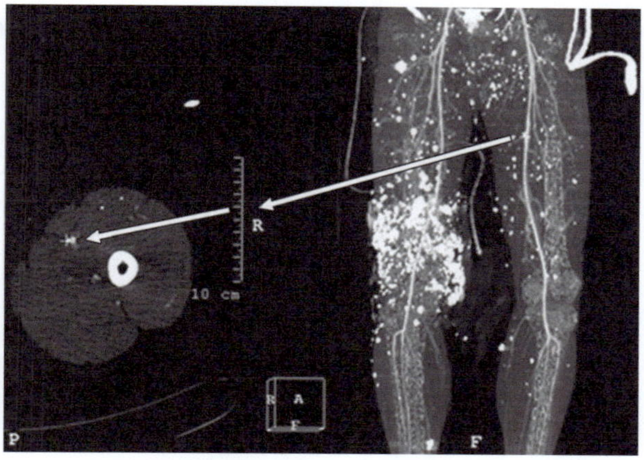

Fig. 9.3 A 27-year-old male soldier with multiple pellets in both legs. Correlation of coronal 3D reconstruction with axial CT-angiography scan allows identification of shrapnel requiring extraction because of threat to the superficial femoral artery (arrows)

During an MCI, the workflow of evaluation should be fast, simple, and standard for all patients. All of these requirements are optimally fulfilled by the CTA examination.

Despite the growing use of CTA as the main diagnostic tool in vascular trauma, there are a few disadvantages that must be brought into consideration. Radiation exposure and the use of iodinated contrast material with the possible allergic reaction or renal toxicity are of concern [20]. Radio-opaque metallic fragments create beam-hardening artifacts impairing CT-angiography [25]. In addition, in CT-angiography there is difficulty in the demonstration of the pedal arteries [20].

9.4.1.5 CTA Signs of Vascular Injury

CTA signs of vascular injury include:

Active contrast extravasation—indicates an ongoing bleeding manifested as a blush of extraluminal contrast material in vicinity to the injured vessel (Fig. 9.4) [20, 24]. Pseudoaneurysm—formation of an extraluminal sac filled with contrast material that is connected by a neck to the injured vessel.

A delayed scan is done in order to distinguish between active bleeding and pseudoaneurym: Active bleeding will usually spread in the delayed scan while pseudoaneurysm will remain in about the same size [24].

Hematoma—a hypodense mass infiltrating the space around an active bleeding or a pseudoaneurysm sac [20]. Hematomas can also be seen without active bleeding or pseudoaneurysm and may vary considerably in size.

Arterio-Venous Fistula—early venous filling on arterial phase, raises suspicion of AVF. Sometimes the exact site and nature of the communication between the artery and vein are not defined by CTA and conventional angiography is recommended [20, 27].

Acute vessel change in caliber or contour—focal stenosis on CTA may indicate the presence of spasm, dissection, or external compression [24]. Irregularity of the vessel wall with lumen narrowing represents wall injury with partial thrombosis [20]. Intraluminal filling defect—can represent thrombus or intimal flap.

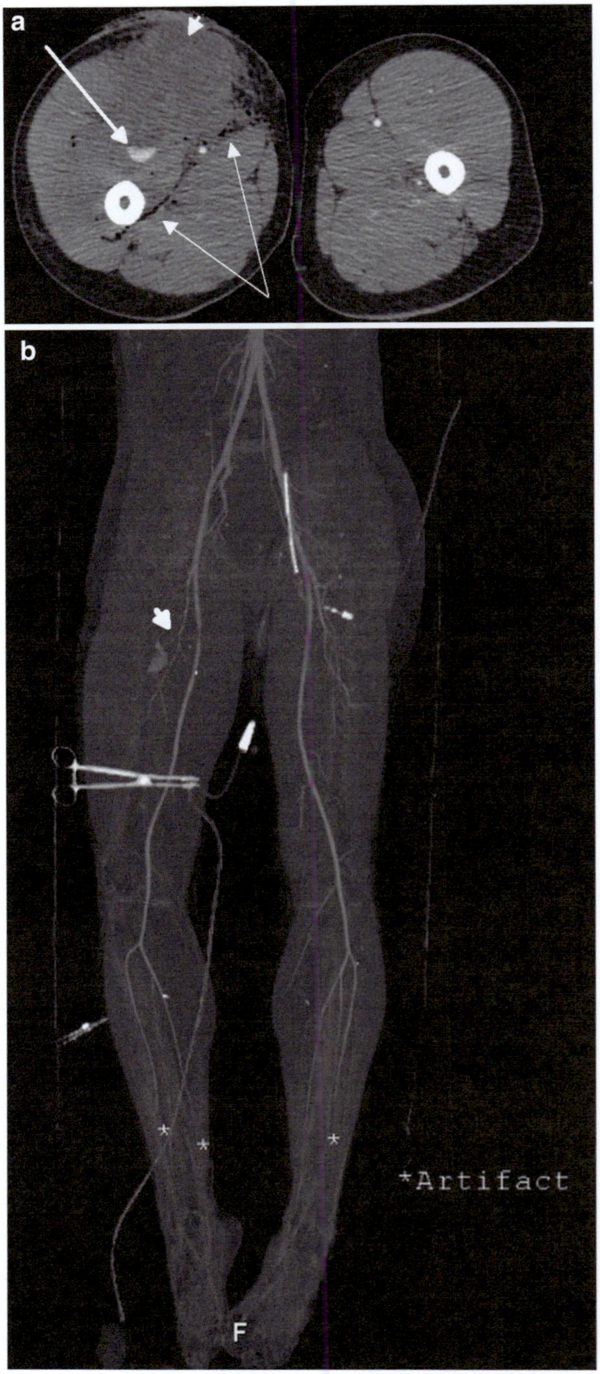

Fig. 9.4 A 21-year-old male soldier with penetrating trauma to the right lower limb. (**a**) CT axial image at the level of the thighs shows a large hematoma (arrowhead) with air bubbles (thin arrows) and a blush of extravasated contrast material (thick arrow). (**b**) 3D-reconstructed image shows torn branches of superficial and deep femoral arteries (arrowhead)

Segmental vessel occlusion may result from transection or complete rupture.

The occlusion may vary in length and distal reconstitution may occur via collaterals [20]. Proximity of shrapnel less than 5 mm from a vessel should raise high suspicion of arterial injury [20].

9.4.1.6 Pitfalls

Occasionally, CT-angiography studies may result in poor diagnostic quality. These are due to improper technique, patient factors, and source artifacts [20, 22]. Poor timing of contrast material bolus resulting in inadequate vessels opacification is one of the most frequent pitfalls.

Injured patient's restlessness due to pain or altered mental status may result in motion artifacts. Inability of a wounded patient to raise his upper extremities overhead when performing upper extremity CT-angiography may lead to streak artifacts from the adjacent torso.

Streak artifacts as a result of metallic fragments in the soft tissues may interfere with the evaluation of an adjacent vessel and prevent exact diagnosis.

9.4.1.7 CTA Technique

A variety of protocols exist, utilizing a multi-detector CT [256, 64, or 16 detectors rows] or a dual energy CT machines. Images are transferred through a local hospital network system to a dedicated work station. Data reconstructions using volume rendering, maximum intensity projection and multiplanar reconstructions are vital in visualization of the arteries. In many institutes, the radiologist and vascular surgeon view the images jointly [20].

Many protocols for a variety of scanners exist. A typical protocol for a 64 slice CTA of the lower extremities usually includes the following parameters: Scan length 1200 mm, slice thickness 2 mm, increment 1 mm, Kv 120, mAs 300, resolution standard, collimation 64× 0.625, pitch 0.703, rotation time 0.5 s. FOV 350 mm, a sharp filter [13], matrix 512, scan time 22–26 s. For contrast injection, an 18 or 20 gauge venous accesses in the antecubital fossa is needed. Injection of contrast media is performed with a dual head injector enabling a "chaser" injection of 40 cc saline. Eighty to one hundred cubic centimeters of contrast media are injected at a rate of 4 cc/s or more.

Delay of scan is usually determined with a bolus tracking protocol with threshold set at 180 HU and a post threshold delay of 3 s. Oral contrast agent is not given.

Scanning is done from the level of the superior mesenteric artery to the feet for a full length lower extremity CTA. A subsequent scan, from the knees to the feet, is added in order to compensate for delayed arterial flow due to vascular injuries. For upper extremity CTA, the injured limb is raised above the head to decrease beam-hardening artifact from the torso and injection of contrast media is done from the contralateral arm. The newer CT scanners offer the ability to integrate peripheral CTA into the routine thoraco-abdominal trauma imaging protocols [20]. Increased acquisition speed of 3–6 s per each body segment allows peripheral CTA and chest or abdominal CTAs to be performed sequentially as needed. This is especially important in combat injury with multiple penetrating and blunt injuries in multilevel sites.

9.4.1.8 Endovascular Treatment

The introduction of CTA in the evaluation of suspected vascular injury has changed the role of conventional arteriography in the traumatized patient. In the authors' institution, conventional arteriography's main role is in the need for endovascular treatment. Another indication is inconclusive CTA due to metal fragments artifacts. Surprisingly, the use of endovascular treatment in MCI is usually very low: In our institute, out of the 849 casualty admitted to the emergency department during the Second Lebanon War only 4 [1%] underwent an endovascular procedure [6] .Yim et al. in a retrospective study from a single trauma center in 2014, reported a 5% usage of endovascular procedures [28] in trauma. Although higher than the author experience, this study was not specifically for an MCI. There is no specific or different recommendation for endovascular treatment in MCI compared to non-MCI vascular trauma and every case should be discussed individually on a case-specific base.

9.4.1.9 Percutaneous Transcatheter Embolization

Embolization in trauma can be used in every site of acute hemorrhage. In the abdomen and pelvis, there are no absolute contraindications to embolization in trauma [29]. Embolization to control active bleeding in the extremities is mainly done in the pelvic vessels and in the proximal branches of the femoral arteries [20]. Compartment syndrome, ischemia, or necrosis is known absolute contraindications for endovascular embolization as these patients should go directly to surgery [29].

When treating a pseudoaneurysm, distal and proximal embolization is important. This method, known as "the sandwich technique," is substantial for obliteration of antegrade and retrograde flow to the pseudoaneurysm [23].

Embolic agents in use include gel foam, coils, and glue. A single agent or a combination may be used [23, 29].

9.4.1.10 Stent/Stent Graft

Indications for stent or stent-graft insertion in the setup of vascular injuries include acute pseudoaneurysm, perforation, AVFs, and dissection [20, 30].

Self-expandable stents are preferable in vascular injury because balloon-mounted stents may cause further damage to the arterial wall. Furthermore, in tortuous vessels, the flexibility of self-expandable stents enables rapid deployment whereas with balloon mounted stents, deployment may be difficult [31].

In general, in the traumatized patient, uncovered stents are indicated in dissections and covered stents in pseudoaneurysms and arterio-venous fistulae [31].

The use of stent graft in urgent aortic trauma, especially blunt trauma has been discussed elsewhere [32]. Although one might assume a thoracic aortic injury takes precedence over other injuries, a patient with a thoracic aortic injury can be observed for several days while additional injuries are treated, as long as appropriate blood pressure controls are observed [32]. This priority rank order fits well within the concept of MCI, e.g., postponing an individual lengthy complex procedure requiring a large number of highly specialized medical personal to a later time when the MCI has ended.

In a large series of treatment with covered stents, in 62 patients with peripheral vascular injuries, White et al., report injuries exclusion success rate of 94% [30].

Piffaretti et al. report ten cases of blunt trauma to peripheral arteries containing pseudoaneurysms, AVFs, dissections, and expanding hematomas, treated successfully with endovascular stents [31]. Limb salvage in this retrospective study was 100%.

Conclusions

In the last decades, there has been a continuous rise in terrorist and other mass casualty incidence. These include motor vehicle accidents, explosions, shootings, earthquakes, and other naturally caused disasters. Thus, every hospital is expected to be prepared for such events and to be trained in managing MCI. This compels every hospital and every department to have pre-planned solutions to the main issues characterizing MCI: the need for an extensive amount of personal, change of the ordinary workflow, and failure of the ordinary cellular phones-based communication.

FAST has an important part in evaluation of all trauma injuries, whether blunt or penetrating, and should be performed on all of them during the resuscitation phase. It is fast, portable, noninvasive, does not involve radiation, and can be integrated into the resuscitation process in the trauma bay without disrupting it.

CT is the modality of choice during an MCI. The protocols used should be simple and standard with a liberal use of whole body protocol in order to avoid time-consuming case-related discussions and reduce the need for repeated visits to the CT suites.

Currently, CTA is the best tool for vascular evaluation in MCI: The advantages of CTA, mainly the speed of the acquisition, the accuracy, and the standardization of the CTA scan, make it an ideal diagnostic tool for vascular imaging in MCI.

Conventional angiography has a very limited role in vascular diagnosis in MCI but has a major role when endovascular treatment is recommended.

References

1. Berger FH, Korner M, Bernstein MP, Sodickson AD, Beenen LF, McLaughlin PD, et al. Emergency imaging after a mass casualty incident: role of the radiology department during training for and activation of a disaster management plan. Br J Radiol. 2016;89:20150984.
2. Ferdia B, Ken L, Steve M, Eric R, Quynh N, Jeffrey R, Bruce L, Joel G. Emergency radiology and mass casualty incidents—report of a mass casualty incident at a level 1 trauma center. Emerg Radiol. 2017;24:47–53.
3. Sosna J, Sella T, Shaham D, Shapira SC, Rivikind A, Bloom A, Libson E. Facing the new threats of terrorism: radiologists' perspectives based on experience in Israel. Radiology. 2005;237:28–36.
4. Victoria SY, Heidi BE, Christine G, Pål AN, Tone E. Radiology response in the emergency department during a mass casualty incident: a retrospective study of the two terrorist attacks on 22 July 2011 in Norway. Eur Radiol. 2017;27:2828–34.

5. Postma ILE, Beenen LFM, Bijlsma TS, Berger FH, Heetveld MJ, Bloemers FW, Goslings JC. Radiological work-up after mass casualty incidents: are ATLS guidelines applicable? Eur Radiol. 2014;24:785–91.
6. Engel A, Soudack M, Ofer A, Nitecki S, Ghersin E, Fischer D, Gaitini DE. Coping with war mass casualties in a hospital under fire: the radiology experience. Am J Roentgenol. 2009;193:1212–21.
7. Brunner J, Rocha TC, Chudgar AA, Goralnick E, Havens JM Raja AS, Sodickson A. The Boston Marathon Bombing: after-action review of the Brigham and Women's Hospital emergency radiology response. Radiology. 2014;273(1):78–87.
8. Gregan J, Balasingam A, Butler A. Radiology in the Christchurch earthquake of 22 February 2011: challenges, interim processes and clinical priorities. J Med Imaging Radiat Oncol. 2016;60:172–81.
9. Poletti PA, Wintermark K, Schnyder P, Becker CD. Traumatic injuries: role of imaging in the management of the polytrauma victim (conservative expectation). Eur Radiol. 2002;12:969–78.
10. Udobi KF, Rodriguez A, Chiu WC, Scalea TM. Role of ultrasonography in penetrating trauma: a prospective clinical study. J Trauma. 2001;50(3):475–9.
11. Miletic D, Fuckar Z, Mraovic B, Dimec D, Mozetic V. Ultrasonography in the evaluation of hemoperitoneum in war casualties. Mil Med. 1999;164:600–3.
12. Sarkisian AE, Khondkarian RA, Amirbekian NM, Bagdasarian NB, Khojayan RL, Oganesian YT. Sonographic screening of mass casualties for abdominal and renal injuries following the 1998 Armenian earthquake. J Trauma. 1991;31(2):247–50.
13. Beck-Razi N, Fischer D, Michaelson M, Engel A, Gaitini D. The utility of focused assessment with Sonography for trauma as a triage tool in multiple casualty incidents during the second Lebanon war. J Ultrasound Med. 2007;26(9):1149–56.
14. Press GM, Miller S. Utility of cardiac tamponade of FAST in blunt trauma. J Emerg Med. 2013;14:9–16.
15. Körner M, Geyer LL, Wirth S, Reiser MF, Linsenmaier U. 64-MDCT in mass casualty incidents: volume image reading boosts radiological workflow. Am J Roentgenol. 2011;197:W399–404.
16. Hare SS, Goddard I, Ward P, Naraghi A, Dick EA. The radiological management of bomb blast injury. Clin Radiol. 2007;62(1):1–9.
17. Singh AK, Goralnick E, George VG, Biddinger PD, Gates J, Sodickson A. Radiologic features of injuries from the Boston Marathon bombing at three hospitals. Am J Roentgenol. 2014;203:235–9.
18. Wolf SJ, Bebarta VS, Bonnett BC, Pons PT, Cantrill SV. Blast injuries. Lancet. 2009;374:405–15.
19. Engel A, Militianu D, Ofer A. Diagnostic imaging in combat trauma. Chapter 7. In: Lerner A, Soudry M, editors. Armed conflict injuries to the extremities. Berlin: Springer; 2011. p. 95–114.
20. Inaba K, Potzman J, Munera F, Mckenny M, Munoz R, Rivas L, Dunham M, DuBose J. Multi-slice CT angiography for arterial evaluation in the injured lower extremity. J Trauma. 2006;60:502–7.
21. Miller-Thomas MM, West OC, Cohen AM. Diagnosing traumatic arterial injury in the extremities with CT angiography: pearls and pitfalls. Radiographics. 2005;25:S133–42.
22. Doody O, Given MF, Lyon SM. Extremities-indications and techniques for treatment of extremity vascular injuries. Injury. 2008;39:1295–303.
23. Madhuripan N, Mehta P, Smolinski SE, Njuguna N. Computed tomography angiography of the extremities in emergencies. Semin Ultrasound CT MR. 2017;38:357–69.
24. Nitecki SS, Karram T, Ofer A, Engel A, Hoffman A. Management of combat vascular injuries using modern imaging: are we getting better? Emerg Med Int. 2013;2013:689473.
25. Soto JA, Munera F, Cardoso N, Guarin O, Medina S. Diagnostic performance of CT angiography in trauma to large arteries of the extremities. J Comput Assist Tomogr. 1999;23(2):188–96.
26. Soto JA, Munera F, Morales C, Lopera JE, Holguin D, Guarin O, Castrillon G, Sanabria A, Garcia G. Focal arterial injuries of the proximal extremities: helical CT arteriography as the initial method of diagnosis. Radiology. 2001;218:188–94.

27. Yim NY, Kim YT, Kim HO, Kim JK, Kang YJ, Park YC, Park CY. Role of interventional radiology in trauma care: retrospective study from single trauma center experience. Am J Emerg Med. 2014 Nov;32(11):1315–8.
28. O'Dell MC, Shah J, Martin JG, Kies D. Emergent endovascular treatment of penetrating trauma: solid organ and extremity. Tech Vasc Interv Radiol. 2017;20:243–7.
29. White R, Krajcer Z, Johnson M, Williams D, Bacharach M, O'malley E. Results of a multicenter trial for the treatment of traumatic vascular injury with a covered stent. J Trauma. 2006;60:1189–95.
30. Piffaretti G, Tozzi M, Lomazzi C, Rivolta N, Caronno R, Lagana D, Carrafiello G. Endovascular treatment for traumatic injuries of the peripheral arteries following blunt trauma. Injury. 2007;38(9):1091–7.
31. Hoffer EK, Forauer AR, Silas AM, Gemery JM. Endovascular stent-graft or open surgical repair for blunt thoracic aortic trauma: systematic review. J Vasc Interv Radiol. 2008;19:1153–64.
32. Kolbeck KJ, Kaufman JA. Endovascular stent grafts in urgent blunt and penetrating thoracic aortic trauma. Semin Intervent Radiol. 2011;28:98–106.

10 Operating Room (OR) Setup, Resource, and Demands

Paola Fugazzola, Matteo Tomasoni, Yoram Kluger,
Luca Ansaloni, and Federico Coccolini

During mass casualty events, a larger portion of victims need emergency surgery compared with victims of conventional trauma. For example, bombing resulted in significantly enhanced use of intensive care, prolonged hospital stay, more surgical interventions, and increased hospital mortality compared to conventional trauma [1]. In this contest, an adequate Operating Room (OR) setup is crucial in order to face a mass casualty event.

There are three main considerations when determining the OR setup:

1. The OR setup should correspond to the OR objective, that should correspond to the overall plan's objective, that is to make an impact on survival rates.
2. OR should be one of the "primary site" in the medical response to a major incident and it is a critical component of surge capacity.
3. OR should be have a quick setup, available 24 h a day and 7 days a week. It shouldn't be affected by the non-office hour.

The main objective of the OR is to identify life-threatening injuries and provide the best treatment (medical and surgical) possible in order to make an impact on survival, at the possible expense of the speed of medical and surgical care of other mild and moderate injuries.

P. Fugazzola · M. Tomasoni · L. Ansaloni · F. Coccolini (✉)
Unit of General and Emergency Surgery, Bufalini Hospital, AUSL Romagna, Cesena, Italy

Y. Kluger
Department of General Surgery, Rambam Health Care Campus, Haifa, Israel

Y. Kluger et al. (eds.), *WSES Handbook of Mass Casualties Incidents Management*, Hot Topics in Acute Care Surgery and Trauma,
https://doi.org/10.1007/978-3-319-92345-1_10

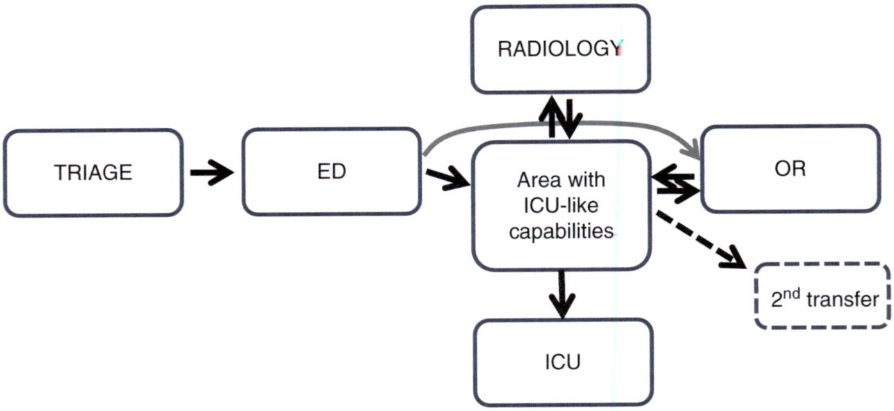

Fig. 10.1 Pathway of severely injured patients

10.1 Pathway of the Severely Injured Patient

In order to best identify and treat patients with life-threatening injuries, severely injured patients should follow an established pathway (Fig. 10.1) that starts with the triage, where the most serious patients are identified. Then patients should be transferred to the Emergency Department (ED). From ED, patients can be transferred directly to the OR or to an area with ICU-like capabilities (e.g., a shock room) where patients undergo first-level diagnostics. From this area, patients are sorted to the OR for emergency surgery, to the radiology department for the second-level diagnostics, or to the ICU-unit.

In different hospitals, this pathway can take different model:

- The ICU-like area could be in the ED (Fig. 10.2a)
- The ICU-like area could be in the ICU (Fig. 10.2b)
- The ICU-like area could be next to the OR (Fig. 10.2c).

In the third model, the ICU-like area could act also as a postoperative recovery unit staffed with ICU-trained nurses, allowing ICU-like monitoring of patients. In the contest of mass casualty events, this model is convenient because it allows to concentrate trauma expertise (surgical specialties, anesthesia/ICU) in a closed working environment of an OR/Recovery Complex.

10.2 Timing of Operation

In addition to identifying which patients need emergency surgery, it is necessary to establish for each patient the urgency of the surgical procedure [2]:

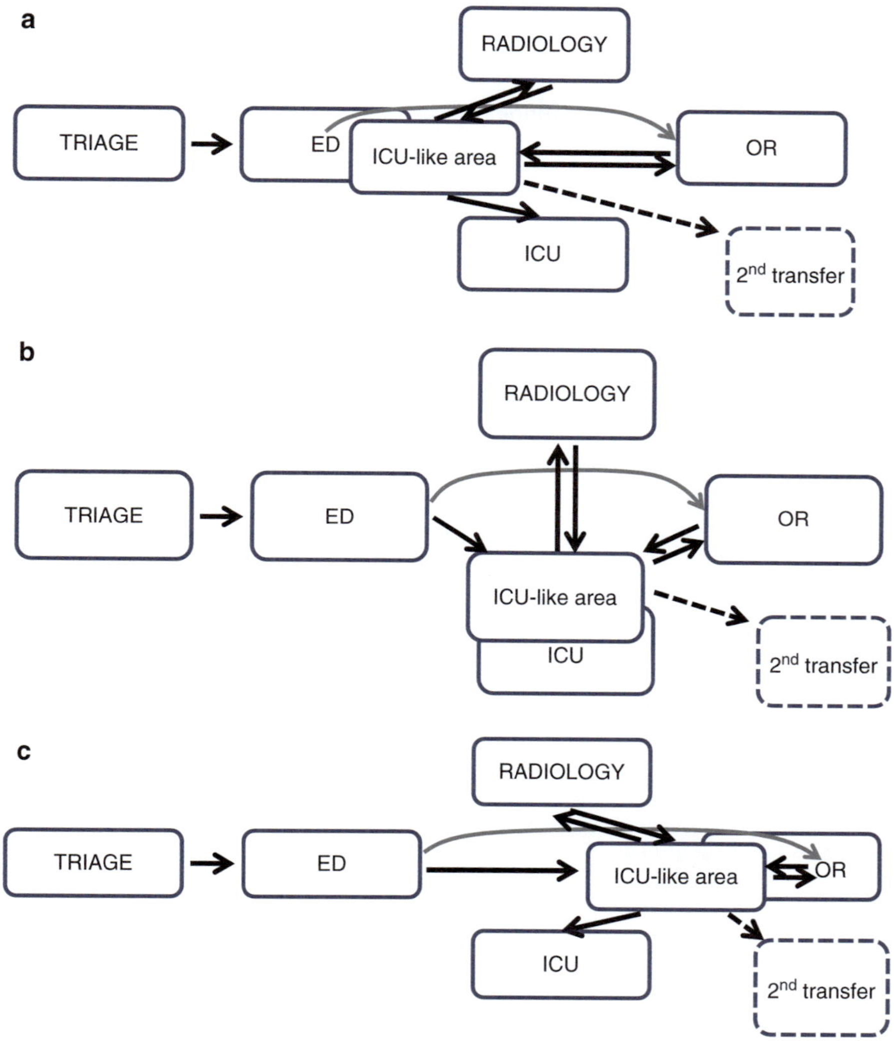

Fig. 10.2 (**a–c**) Different models of pathway for severely injured patients

1. Immediate for unstable patient in need of immediate lifesaving operation.
2. Urgent in stable patient with life-threatening pathology, whose operation should be started as early as possible (<2 h).
3. High priority in stable patients with life-threatening pathology whose operation may be delayed no more than 3–4 h.
4. Delayed in stable patients with injuries for which surgery can be delayed for several hours, such as limb-threatening injuries (4–12 h).
5. Non-urgent for stable patients whose surgery can be delayed beyond 12 h without untoward complications.

In a work on four hundred patients admitted in 19 mass casualty events following bombing incidents, 39 (9.3%) patients had an injury severity score ≥16 and of 68 patients who were operated, 28 (6.6%) were in need of either immediate, urgent, or high-priority operations (constituting over half of severely injured patients) [2].

Conclusions

- During mass casualty events, the hospital should expect at least 1 of 10 victims will suffer from a life-threatening injury and half of these will need an emergency operation.
- Hospitals should consider the "OR/Recovery Complex" model with an ICU-like area near the OR in order to create a closed environment with ability to concentrate all those with trauma experience; this allows triage of surgical priorities, imaging priorities, and second transfer.
- Remember to make an impact on survival, most if not all the initial resources should be allocated to the diagnosis of those severely injured. Those experienced in trauma are the most important resource that can make an impact on survival of severely injured victims.

References

1. Kluger Y, Peleg K, Daniel-Aharonson L, Mayo A, Israeli Trauma Group. The special injury pattern in terrorist bombings. J Am Coll Surg. 2004;199(6):875–9.
2. Ashkenazi I, Turégano-Fuentes F, Einav S, Kessel B, Alfici R, Olsha O. Pitfalls to avoid in the medical management of mass casualty incidents following terrorist bombings: the hospital perspective. Eur J Trauma Emerg Surg. 2014;40(4):445–50. https://doi.org/10.1007/s00068-014-0403-x. Epub 2014 May 1.

11 Intensive Care Unit (ICU): Resources and Demands

Andrew J. Kamien, Christopher S. Davis, and Marc A. de Moya

11.1 Introduction

In recent times, the medical profession has been challenged by a variety of mass casualty events (MCEs) of both natural and man-made disasters. Intensive Care Unit (ICU) management is crucial to successful treatment during an MCE, as a significant proportion of these patients (2.5–34%) will require critical care [1].

Delivery of critical care has its own specific needs and therefore its own vulnerabilities, and although each MCE is unique (type of disaster, patient casualty size, current critical care capabilities, duration of casualty-generating circumstance) there are commonly encountered challenges for all MCEs. Despite the variety of these challenges, some have advocated for an approach of "standardized process and customized response" [2]. It is necessary that all ICUs have a general MCE plan in place that defines the "realistic hospital capacity," which is the admitting capacity as determined by available medical/surgical resources and number of trauma teams [3]. Recommendations from the Task Force for Mass Critical Care Summit state that all ICUs should be able to effectively triple their capacities and maintain their own care for a minimum of 10 days before expecting external assistance [4]. Therefore, pre-planned organization is key, as past events have demonstrated that this population requires critical care for approximately 10–21 days [5, 6].

Several lessons have been learned over the last several decades from various MCEs. We will review recommendations that stem from those events, as well as guidelines for some of the commonly encountered needs, while providing recommendations for methods to triage care in the face of shortages. We discuss three major categories of need: intervention and equipment, staff, and space, and finalize our review with an emphasis on triage and resource allocation [1].

A. J. Kamien · C. S. Davis · M. A. de Moya (✉)
Medical College of Wisconsin/Froedtert Hospital, Milwaukee, WI, USA
e-mail: mdemoya@mcw.edu

Y. Kluger et al. (eds.), *WSES Handbook of Mass Casualties Incidents Management*, Hot Topics in Acute Care Surgery and Trauma,
https://doi.org/10.1007/978-3-319-92345-1_11

11.2 Interventions and Equipment

Emergency Mass Critical Care (EMCC) includes the interventions listed in Table 11.1. In addition to these interventions, the ICU must also have available sufficient materials to make delivery of critical care possible.

Mechanical ventilation is unique to the ICU environment, and a potential limitation, as approximately 70–80% of those patients in critical condition require the assistance of a mechanical ventilator [5, 7, 8]. In some series, 37% of those who are critically ill will require mechanical ventilation for greater than 7 days [5]. Most institutions carry only a minimal number of reserve ventilators at any time. Redistribution or rental of these machines could potentially expand the capacity for one institution at a given time, but the logistics of this may be prohibitive. Additionally, dependent upon the nature of the MCE and how widespread it may reach (bio-terrorism, nation-wide pandemic), only a finite number of mechanical ventilators are available in this country. The most optimistic estimates are 35 ventilators available for every 100,000 people, meaning that patient need may overcome potential supply [9].

Given these shortages, various alternatives to traditional mechanical ventilation have been suggested, such as substitution with noninvasive positive pressure ventilation (when able), utilization of operating room anesthesia machines, and modification of a single machine to treat multiple patients [1]. Each of these has its own potential strengths and weaknesses; however, all efforts should be made to maximize the mechanical ventilation capacity. Ideally, ventilation equipment should have the following qualities: (1) be able to oxygenate and ventilate most pediatric and adult patients with either significant airflow obstruction or acute respiratory distress syndrome; (2) be able to function with low-flow oxygen and without high-pressure medical gas; (3) accurately deliver a prescribed minute ventilation when patients are not breathing spontaneously; and (4) have sufficient alarms to alert the operator to apnea, circuit disconnect, low gas source, low battery, and high peak airway pressures.

Many of the other medical equipment and supplies in the ICU are otherwise classified as consumable products, and therefore an MCE would make any unit vulnerable to shortages, especially since most hospitals operate under the "just in time" supply model and are reliant upon re-stocking for any acute needs. Oxygen is one

Table 11.1 Emergency Mass Critical Care (EMCC) interventions

1. Mechanical ventilation
2. Intravenous fluids
3. Vasopressors
4. Antibiotics, or other disease specific treatments
5. Sedation and analgesia
6. Standard critical care prophylactic measures
7. Optimal therapeutics and interventions, such as continuous renal replacement therapy and means of nutrition

From Devereaux AV et al. Chest 2008

Table 11.2 Medications for emergency medical critical care

Sedation and analgesia	Benzodiazepines
	Opioids
	Succinylcholine
	Non-depolarizing paralytic agent
Bronchodilators	Anticholinergics and beta-agonists
Crystalloids	0.9% NaCl or Lactated Ringers Solution
Vasopressors	Institution preferences
Antimicrobials	Infectious Disease Society of America's Guidelines
Anticoagulants	Institutional preferences
Hormones	Insulin
	Hydrocortisone

such consumable commonly stored in large bulk in a liquid form; yet, this can be of critical need in the setting of increased demand and/or damaged storage.

As re-stocking of supplies is not likely to be feasible during an MCE, any traditionally consumable devices should be disinfected with the purpose of re-use when applicable [9]. For those items that re-use is not an option, accurate stocking and knowledge of consumables (Table 11.2) should be inspected with some regularity [10]. Strategies to re-stock and re-supply have otherwise been described by Lynn et al. by way of specifically designated ICU carts listed in Table 11.3, each with enough supplies expected to care for 20 patients [11].

11.3 Staff

ICUs routinely face staffing shortages, and although staff shortages have not been a major issue in past MCEs, the potential remains. Adequate staffing for ICU care encompasses not only the nursing and physicians, but also other medical staff (respiratory technicians, radiology technicians, lab technicians, nursing assistants, and clerks), as well as other support staff (electricians, maintenance workers, and security) [11].

Dependent upon the type of disaster, absenteeism can be expected to range between 10 and 60%. Potential risks for absenteeism include disasters of a prolonged duration and those that have concrete effects on the personal lives of staff (e.g., school and day-care closures, elder-care issues) or those with hypothetical risks, as bio-events may cause staff to fail to report for duty out of fear of becoming themselves or spreading infection to their families [9]. Indeed, ICU staff may be of particular risk during the case of an MCE. During the sarin subway poisoning in Japan in 1995 for example, nearly one-fourth of the hospital staff had exposure, which disproportionately affected nursing (39.3% of nursing assistants and 26.5% of nurses), as well as the ICU staff specifically (38.7% of staff) [12].

Given the risks and demands of staffing shortages, one must generate the maximum reserve during an incident, and the following rules should be extended

Table 11.3 List of supplies for ICU Cart (20 patients)

1. Two red emergency crash carts
2. Two hospital intubation/airway trays
3. One thoracotomy tray
4. Two 28-Fr chest tubes
5. Two 32-Fr chest tubes
6. Sutures: one box 2.O silk straight needle
7. Sutures: one box O silk straight and curved needle
8. Twenty blood pressure cuffs (with continuous noninvasive capability)
9. Twenty monitors with EKG and pulse oximetry
10. Forty sterile gowns, 20 sterile drapes, sterile gloves (one box each of size 7, 7-1/2, and 8)
11. Nonsterile gloves: two boxes each of small, medium, and large. Caps and masks: one box each
12. Gauze 4 × 4-inch (four boxes), 8 × 12-inch (four boxes), and 2 × 2-inch (two boxes)
13. Syringes (3, 5, 10, and 20 mL): three boxes each
14. Nasogastric tubes: 10 each
15. Suction capabilities for 20 beds, minimum 2 per bedside
16. Thirty suction canisters with tubing and extensions
17. Central lines: 8–9.0 Fr-introducers, 8- to 20-cm triple lumen catheter
18. Peripheral IVs: 10- to 20-gauge, 10- to 18-gauge
19. Fifteen IV start kits
20. Tape: silk tape, 3-in and 5-in, 10 rolls each
21. Restraints: 15 pairs
22. IV pumps: 20
23. IV regulation Gtt tubing: 25 each
24. IV primary pump tubing: 25 each
25. Blood tubing: 15 each
26. Normal saline (0.9%) 1-L bags, 40 each
27. Lactated Ringer's, 1-L bags, 40 each
28. D5LR 20 bags
29. D51/2NS, 40 mEq KCL/L, 20 bags each
30. Lab tubes: ABG syringes 100, tiger tops one box, purple/blue/green tops one box each
31. Drugs: Morphine 4 mg × 50, morphine 10 mg × 50, midazolam 5 mg × 50, propofol 100-mL bottles × 10, lorazepam 2 mg × 60, haloperidol (multidose bottle) (10)
32. Potassium 20 mEq (10), Potassium 10 mEq (50)
33. Magnesium 1 g (10)
34. Nitroglycerine, 25-mg bottles (4)
35. Furosemide, 20 mg (10)
36. Ranitidine, 50 mg (40)
37. Nicardipine, 50 mg (2)
38. Labetalol: four (4) bottles
39. Intubation bronchoscope on standby
40. Twenty patient charts
41. Bag-valve-mask (20)
42. Pressure bags (liter size) (15)
43. Oxygen flow meters (20)
44. Pleura vacs (3)
45. Alcohol swabs
46. Yankauer suction (20)
47. Chlorhexidine and betadine five (5) each
48. Stopcocks (40)
49. Tracheotomy tray (1) with size 8 and 6 shiley cuffed tubes

universally to all staffing units: (1) postponement of any vacation; (2) extension of work hours; and (3) staggering the recall of off-duty staff and instituting sleep schedules to mitigate fatigue [1]. In the wake of these catastrophic and emotionally charged events, it is a natural tendency to come to aid immediately. However, keeping in mind that these events often persist for days and even weeks, it is incumbent to schedule shifts so that one's workforce is not exhausted after the first 24 h.

In regard to the prevention of staffing shortages from biologic events, roles for decontamination and personal protective equipment (PPE) are required. There needs to be complete adherence to infection control and utilization of PPE, including gowns and gloves, and also to ensure there is regular fitting for respirators such as the N-95. Though continuous monitoring is not practical, it is unsafe to assume that adherence to PPE practices is complete. Accordingly, periodic monitoring is suggested to maximize early identification and to triage those at risk [12].

There are position-specific recommendations for staff as well. MCEs create an immediate need for critical care nursing, so much so that the United States government's National Disaster Management System maintains Disaster Medical Assistant Teams (DMATs) that are ready for deployment, which include ICU nurses. Other options include recruitment of ICU staff from other non-ICU environments, recruitment of nurses from Federal Emergency Management Agency or locum agencies (in addition to DMAT), maintaining interim refresher courses for former ICU nurses to keep up their skills in the event of an emergency, emergency credentialing, and increasing the nursing-to-patient ratio [10].

Critical care is also reliant upon a significant number of ancillary staff, and, although recruitment strategies have not been described, minimizing workload of the support staff has a clear role. For instance, a shift in practice for laboratory testing practice has been advocated, thereby minimizing unnecessary tests to free up time for more critical lab tests that yield actionable information. Additionally, minimizing need for transport out of the ICU (e.g., for specialized imaging) will allow the nursing staff to remain in the ICU and decrease the demands of transport staff and respiratory therapists, as most critical care patients are intubated [1].

Groups have suggested that there will be a demand of intensivist-physicians, as well during an MCE. Past events have demonstrated the inefficient use of resources by those over-extending their realm of practice in a critical care setting. Therefore, to maximize the amount of potential care provided by ICU staff, critical care staff should oversee non-critical care providers. This can be performed in a two-tier system, as non-intensivists perform the general medical care of a small group of critically ill patients with an intensivist managing the acute emergencies and overseeing a group of these non-intensivists. This means of organization extends the capabilities of a single intensivist and should prevent non-intensivists from potentially misusing a finite amount of resources [10]. In this context, pre-printed protocols may be of assistance to the non-intensivists in managing care [2].

Finally, lessons can be learned from the London bombings of July 2005 regarding staffing and organization to execute cares. The Royal London Hospital (RLH) utilized a dedicated clerk that was responsible for creating and constantly updating a worksheet that listed each individual patient, their injuries, pending and completed diagnostic workup, as well as pended and completed operations. This kept information centralized and updated for the intensivists to most efficiently manage care. This became crucial as the internal phone systems and mobile networks both went down during the attacks, and the RLH utilized runners as the best method of properly disseminating the most up-to-date information. Lastly, another example from RLH that can be modeled as it relates to staffing is the use of multidisciplinary teams in patient care. This ensured that decisions were being made with the most updated information possible. Ultimately, the care teams found it necessary to conduct the multidisciplinary meetings at a central location [7].

11.4 Space

Critical care is unique in that there are limited areas where it can be provided on a routine basis outside of current critical care designations. In the case of an MCE, some non-medical areas (schools, gymnasiums, hotels, sports fields) can be utilized to provide basic care [9]. Given the specific needs of electricity, oxygen, suctioning, medical gases, monitoring equipment, and the physical space required to house these items, critical care is also limited to specific areas in the hospital. Accordingly, knowledge of where all back-up power and emergency outlets are located is encouraged, and plans to have generator as back-up should be in place.

In the absence of an MCE, most hospitals and level-1 trauma centers operate at or near capacity. The need for potential space is further limited in the case of a pandemic or bio-terrorism. For example, during the severe acute respiratory syndrome outbreak of Toronto in 2005, approximately one-third of the ICU space was closed due to quarantine requirements which lasted 12–14 days [13].

Past strategies to maximize space have included the cancellation of all elective operations and freeing up currently used space in the hospital, which can increase hospital capacity up to 20% [10]. During the Madrid bombing of 2004, local hospitals were able to discharge 161 patients within 2 h, and all stable ICU patients were transferred to the floor to make room for new ICU admissions [5]. Surge capacity can be also be expanded within the ICU, and EMCC can be extended to the post-anesthesia care unit, emergency department, step-down units, procedural suites, and telemetry units [1]. Knowledge of the potential capabilities of a unit can prove invaluable. During the nightclub fire of Rhode Island in 2003, a 22-bed ICU was quickly expanded to a capacity of 34 beds [6].

11.5 Triage and Resource Allocation

Despite all planning efforts, however, ICU providers will ultimately find themselves in a triage setting when faced with an MCE. This requires a paradigm shift in care, from the application of unlimited resources for the greatest good of everyone to the allocation of limited resources for the greatest good of the greatest number of casualties [10].

The triage process should ideally begin at time-point zero immediately after the event and before any patients arrive at the hospital, as there have been previously documented linear relationships with over-triage and critical mortality, suggesting that utilization of resources by non-critically ill patients compromise future patient care [1]. Therefore, in the wake of a massive influx of patients to the hospital, triage should be performed by senior physician at the emergency department or hospital entrance. Early involvement of ICU staff should be encouraged for their knowledge and expertise in managing acutely ill patients and in anticipation of where potential delays in patient care and transfer might occur.

Dependent upon the demands of the MCE and resources available, resource allocation and even reallocation may be eventually necessary. Recommendations for allocation of scarce resources in mass casualty events have been provided by the Task Force for Critical Care Summit Meeting from January 2007. Critical care will be rationed under the following tenets: (1) all efforts at augmentation have been exceeded; (2) limitations on who is deemed critical will be proportional to the acute shortfall in resources; (3) rationing of critical care will occur uniformly, be transparent, and abide by objective medical criteria; (4) rationing should apply equally to withholding and withdrawing life-sustaining treatments based on the principle that withholding and withdrawing care are ethically equivalent; and (5) patients not eligible for critical care will continue to receive supportive medical or palliative therapy [14].

Potential triggers for initiation of a triage algorithm include shortages of the previously described cores of critical care: lack of equipment, lack of infrastructure, lack of staffing/specialty care, and the inability to transfer patients to another medical facility. Following establishment of needing to initiate rationing of care, each individual patient needs to be investigated by inclusion and exclusion criteria. For inclusion criteria, patients must require active critical care interventions; in other words, there is no place for "observation" ICU cares. Patients meet exclusion criteria if they have a very high risk of mortality, little likelihood of long-term survival, and a correspondingly low likelihood of benefit from critical care resources. To objectively measure each potential need, patients may have a $\geq$80% risk of death if the following criteria are met: highest sequential organ failure assessment (SOFA) score $\geq$ 15 at any time; mean SOFA $\geq$ 5 for at least 5 days and with a trend that is either rising or flat; or patients with six or more organ failures at any time. Additional exclusion criteria, as they relate to chronic illness, include end-stage congestive heart failure, end-stage chronic obstructive pulmonary disease, and terminal liver disease. SOFA scores are to be calculated daily and patients should be constantly reevaluated for potential reallocation of care. In the absence of exclusion criteria, prioritization may need to occur. Further potential need for reallocation of resources away from certain patients can be inferred if the following criteria are met: (1) those with the highest SOFA score and/or a trend that is either rising or flat; (2) having a high degree of inpatient acuity with a poor chance for survival and/or a likely long duration of need of resources; (3) a moderate degree of acuity but a prolonged duration of critical care resources; and (4) severe underlying critical care illness that, in conjunction with any of the above factors, leads a decision-maker to feel the prognosis is poor and/or the patient's likely duration of care resources is prolonged. For those who meet criteria for reallocation of care, it is required that these individuals continue to receive palliative care [14].

Conclusions

Medical decision-making for disaster planning is complex, and the ICU is no different as it must be able to function independently with its own vulnerabilities in the context of the hospital as a whole. It is necessary that each ICU provides its own plan of action for a potential MCE. Attention to the unique categories that we have discussed will provide a framework for the identification of needs and vulnerabilities of an ICU, while providing guidance for triage situations and the potential reallocation of care.

References

1. Corcoran SP, et al. Critical care management of major disasters: a practical guide to disaster preparation in the intensive care unit. J Intensive Care Med. 2012;27(1):3–10.
2. Parker MM. Critical care and disaster management. Crit Care Med. 2006;34(3 Suppl):S52–5.
3. Hirshberg A, Holcomb JB, Mattox KL. Hospital trauma care in multiple-casualty incidents: a critical review. Ann Emerg Med. 2001;37:647–52.
4. Devereaux AV, et al. Summary of suggestions from the Task Force for Mass Critical Care Summit, January 26–27, 2007. Chest. 2008;133:1S–7S.
5. Ceballos, et al. 11 March 2004: The terrorist bomb explosions in Madrid, Spain – an analysis of the logistics, injuries sustained and clinical management of casualties treated at the closest hospital. Crit Care. 2005;9:104–11.
6. Mahoney EJ, Harrington DT, Biffl WL, Metzger J, Oka T, Cioffi WG. Lessons learned from a nightclub fire: institutional disaster preparedness. J Trauma. 2005;58:487–91.
7. Shirley PJ, Mandersloot G. Clinical review: the role of the intensive care physician in mass casualty incidents: planning, organisation, and leadership. Crit Care. 2008;12:214.
8. Vered Avidan V, et al. Civilian hospital response to a mass casualty event: the role of the intensive care unit. J Trauma. 2007;62:1234–9.
9. Christian MD, et al. Definitive care the critically ill during disaster: Current capabilities and limitations: from a Task Force for Mass Critical Care summit meeting, January 26-27, 2007, Chicago, IL. Chest. 2008;133(5 Suppl):8S–17S.
10. Mahoney EJ, et al. Mass-casualty incidents: how does an ICU prepare. J Intensive Care Med. 2008;23(4):219–35.
11. Lynn M, Gurr D, Memon A, Kaliff J. Management of conventional mass casualty incidents: ten commandments for hospital planning. J Burn Care Res. 2006;27(5):649–58.
12. Sumie Okumura S, et al. Clinical review: Tokyo – protecting the health care worker during a chemical mass casualty event: an important issue of continuing relevance. Crit Care. 2005;9:397–400.
13. Hawryluck L, Lapinsky SE, Stewart TE. Clinical review: SARS – lessons in disaster management. Crit Care. 2005;9(4):384–9.
14. Devereaux AV, et al. Definitive care for the critically ill during a disaster: a framework for allocation of scarce resources in mass critical care. From a Task Force for Mass Critical Care Summit Meeting, January 26–27, 2007, Chicago, IL. Chest. 2008;133:51S–66S.

12 The Pediatric Patient in MCI

Adam Lee Goldstein and Dror Soffer

12.1 Introduction

Despite the demographic minority of children in any given population, mass casualty incidents (MCI) often impact areas with a high concentration of children, such as schools and recreational events. Even those MCI primarily involving children are initially met by healthcare workers trained to provide care for adults (from the first-response team to the specialty physicians), as well as an infrastructure designed for triaging, transporting, and treating adult patients.

In 2016, children (age 0–14 years) comprised 19% of the population of the United States. Worldwide, the countries with the lowest percentage of children (13%) included Japan, Germany, and Bosnia. The countries with the highest percent of children (48%) included Angola, Chad, and Uganda [1].

Despite comprising about 10% of all ambulance calls/transport in the developed world, pediatric patients have been found to have a higher death rate than adults after a traumatic event in the pre-hospital setting [2]. Much of this discrepancy has been attributed to a lack of preparedness on all levels of care. During disasters, age has proven inversely related to likelihood of morbidity and mortality [3]. On a daily basis (in non-MCI situations), 89% of emergency room visits by children are to non-pediatric hospitals or pediatric emergency centers. Of these care centers, only 6% were found to be adequately prepared for pediatric patients [4]. Adding the extreme strain of an MCI to this chronically underprepared system creates an untenable situation for pediatric patients. With MCI involving a large number of casualties, the hospital's emergency center then becomes a place of "first response," as victims flood the hospital with or without pre-hospital care or triage.

A. L. Goldstein (✉)
The Department of General Surgery, Tel Aviv Sourasky Medical Center, Tel Aviv, Israel

D. Soffer
Yitzhak Rabin Trauma Division, Tel Aviv Sourasky Medical Center, Tel Aviv, Israel

Y. Kluger et al. (eds.), *WSES Handbook of Mass Casualties Incidents Management*, Hot Topics in Acute Care Surgery and Trauma,
https://doi.org/10.1007/978-3-319-92345-1_12

Current disaster-planning estimates that, for every one critical patient in need of acute care, there will be five "unaffected" patients seeking treatment [5]. With compliant adults, it is easy for care providers to give instructions and continue treating those in need. In contrast, with the pediatric population, even the "unaffected" will require a significant level of care, resources, and manpower due to the patients' developmental limitations (most particularly with infants) and their vulnerability to further significant physical and emotional injury. In addition to the baseline complex infrastructure formed and activated in a rushed time-frame, additional specialized medical training, equipment, and expertise are needed to deal with issues pertaining to the diverse pediatric population. This may range from advanced neonatal care, to organizing reunification efforts, to feeding and/or comforting distressed infants. All of these needs are vital and, if ignored, may compromise or hinder all aspects of the relief effort—from the first triage minutes after the MCI to definitive care and the affected community's post-MCI recuperation efforts. Therefore, the needs of the pediatric population must be anticipated and planned for during both the development of pre-emptive protocols and the acute response to the MCI.

Even when a healthcare system conducts MCI drills, most do not include pediatric patients [6]. Critical differences exist in the anatomy and physiology of adults and children (with additional differences between infant, toddlers, and children), and by not understanding these differences in pathophysiology and practicing procedures specific for pediatrics there will continue to be preventable and unacceptable higher rates in morbidity and mortality. One study surveying 1932 randomly selected ambulance services across the United States showed that only 18.8% had any sort of protocol outlining a pediatric patient plan during an MCI, and only 31.8% had a response plan for an MCI at a school [7]. This study also demonstrated that only 25.7% of the services reported any sort of collaboration or cooperation with the local school district, and only 12.3% worked together with a pediatrician on a regular basis to help establish pre-hospital protocols and training. In multiple studies, it has been demonstrated that, on all levels of response and treatment, both equipment/supplies and pre-emptive plans to deploy the necessary personnel are markedly lacking, including everything from a sufficiency of pediatricians and pediatric surgeons to correctly sized blood pressure cuffs, IVs, and pediatric doses of lifesaving medicines. These deficiencies are the current norm, despite children being the most physically, physiologically, and mentally at risk during violent or natural disasters [8].

This chapter will focus on the MCI-related pediatric patient and review the physiological, emotional, and logistical challenges involved when dealing with this population during an MCI. We will conclude with concrete recommendations based on a review of the literature and personal experiences. It must be recalled that, under the umbrella of "MCI," there are an increasing variety of possible mechanisms and therefore, a greater heterogeneity injuries. Nevertheless, we will focus on principles that may be relevant for any sort of MCI involving the pediatric patient.

12.1.1 Organization and Triage

The first step in effective treatment for the pediatric patient, may it be in the field or hospital, is allocating appropriate resources and mobilizing specific manpower for the pediatric population and current situation. This includes pediatric nurses, neonatologists, pediatricians, pediatric intensivists, pediatric anesthesiologists, and pediatric surgeons (including the relevant surgical specialties orthopedics and neurosurgery). A specific communication network and protocol must be in place, practiced, and appropriately activated when there are injured children and pediatric specialists are needed to be mobilized quickly. These pediatric specialists must be accessible. Which means that at a time of disaster/MCI, when cellular networks are usually jammed, a pager or alternative communication system must be available and activated [9].

Once first response and treatment begins, the physical location of the casualties grouped by age group (pediatric & adult) will help simplify the treatment efforts by organizing the pediatric supplies and focusing the pediatric specialist around the pediatric patients. Pediatric supplies should be marked with a specific color in order to avoid confusion and rapid access. The medical team caring for the pediatric patients must be clearly marked with a colored over-shirt/jersey/vest that identifies them as the pediatric team. The head of the pediatric triage should be a senior pediatric surgeon who is the sole line of contact with the officer running the entire rescue/treatment effort. If a pediatric expert is not immediately accessible, the triage officer at scene will be the initial healthcare provider prioritizing the adult and pediatric patients. Readily available and accessible pediatric/age-specific laminated cards and protocols (ranging from first-response treatments, triage, medicine dosage, and definitive care) may be lifesaving during the stress and disorder of the acute event, and vital before a pediatric specialist is able to take control of the operation.

Certain triage methods for pediatrics have been better studied and proven than others. The most widely accepted triage method developed for adults and pediatrics is the SALT (Sort, Assess, Lifesaving intervention, Transport) method, which was created by an expert panel in 2008 charged with recommending one universal "overarching" triage method for the United States capable of being studied and validated [10]. Despite the evolution of this universal triage system, JumpSTART, a pediatric triage system published in 2002, continues to be highly recommended and (theoretically) used for pediatric patients during an MCI. JumpSTART is a modification of the START triage system for adults (replaced by SALT) which takes into account the unique pathophysiology of children (specifically ages 1–8 years) by including rescue breaths for the pulseless child, based on the fact that most cardiac arrest in children is due to hypoxia and respiratory failure. When comparing SALT and JumpSTART, there were no major differences in accuracy between the two [11]. An expert panel focusing on the triage of the pediatric patient in Israel recommended the use of JumpSTART for our EMS teams [12] (Fig. 12.1). A study from South Africa compared different triage methods for pediatric trauma patients (not related

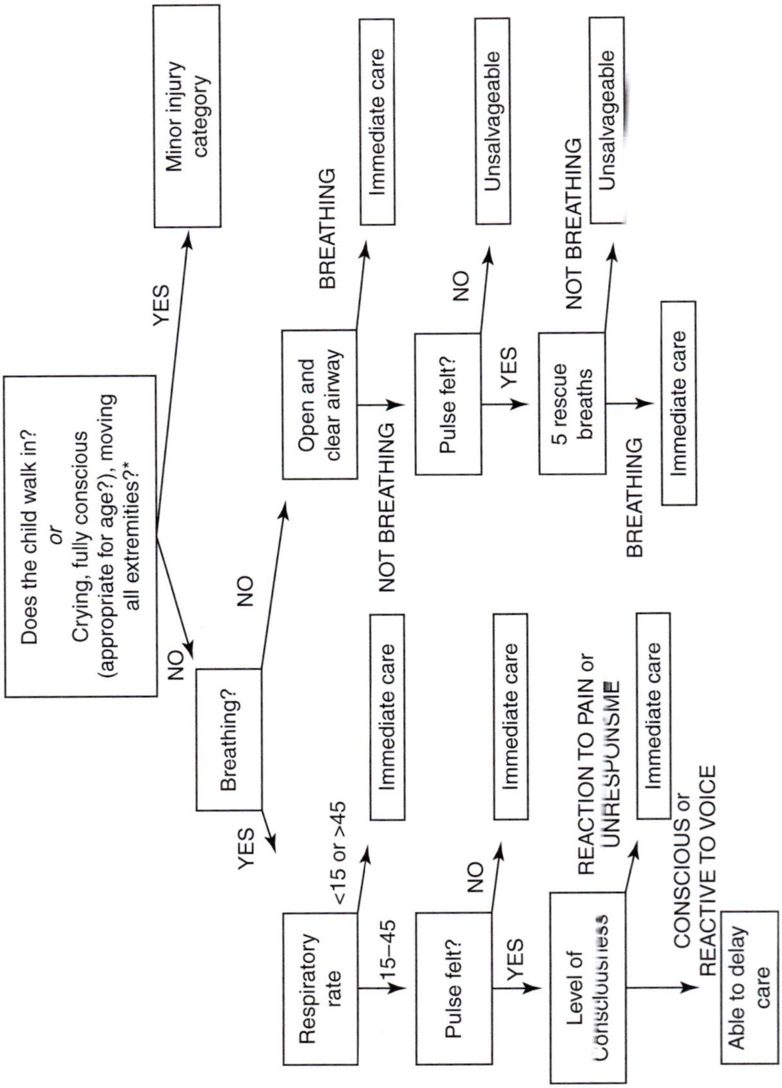

Fig. 12.1 The JumpSTART triage algorithm

to an MCI), assessing established pediatric triage methods from the UK (the pediatric triage tape), Australia (Careflight), and JumpSTART. They found that JumpSTART was less sensitive to serious injuries and recommended against its use [13]. Nevertheless, JumpSTART has recently been found to be the most currently utilized method in the United States among EMS providers [14]. Although JumpSTART has been found adequate, even the first decision point of if the patient is "walking" may be dangerously misleading to the untrained provider with regard to infants and children before walking age.

Not only for diagnostics, but also for triage, ultrasound (US) has been found to be a valuable tool in the field and hospital during traumatic events [15]. Especially in children, due to their small size, their sensitivity of US is increased and may be utilized for a wide range of diagnostic or therapeutic purposes—from detecting free fluid in the abdomen, pneumothorax/effusion or pericardial effusion to assisting with IV access. Especially for pediatric, it is practical and useful to utilize US as a triage tool, with all patients undergoing an extended focal assessment with sonography for trauma (E/FAST) in order to help identify children with critical injuries and need for surgery [16]. According to the JumpSTART algorithm, the US may be performed before the child is categorized as minor injury or after the initial trauma survey of airway, breathing, and circulation to those initially categorized as critical to help identify primary injuries.

A form of triage will occur in both the field and the hospital. An important aspect of triage when preparing for pediatric injuries is coordination with level 1 pediatric trauma centers. The availability of specialized pediatric care is directly related to outcomes. Depending on the location of the event and distance from a pediatric trauma center, an emphasis on accurate and well-thought-out transport in order to get the pediatric patients to the appropriate care may be more immediately important than the triage procedure, which can take place more efficiently and accurately at the appropriate trauma center [17]. Any hospital, pediatric or not, must know how to prepare to receive a MCI. This entails a designated team to initiate the immediate preparations for the MCI, and protocols that are routinely drilled with the entire hospital staff. The emergency room and trauma bays must be rapidly emptied of all non-urgent patients not involved in the MCI, whom are transported to the wards without further workup [18]. For the non-children's hospitals, once children have been identified as victims, a designated area is made for the pediatric teams (as mentioned above), with their own triage and resuscitation area.

Applying the overall goals and philosophy of triage to an MCI involving children raises many ethical questions. One may argue that children should be given priority (when compared to an adult with the same category of injury) because of the potential work-force years that a child has compared to an adult. Children also provoke a greater emotional response within the triage officer, complicating the triage procedure and creating a bias and advantage toward children compared to injured adults [13].

12.1.2 The Anatomical and Physiological Differences in Pediatric Patients

From the airway, hemodynamics, and definitive operative or critical care, a child's differences from adult patients are significant and must be understood in order to optimize treatment and chances of survival in both the pre-hospital and hospital setting. Lack of preparedness during the resulting chaos of an MCI will have a negative impact not only on the lives of the pediatric patients, but on the entire rescue operation and overall outcome.

Compared to an adult, the anatomy of an infant or child's body is more vulnerable to injury. Their internal chest and abdominal organs are larger, closer together, and less well protected by skeletal structures and musculature [19], leaving them more susceptible to multi-visceral injury. Especially in infants and small children, the head-to-body ratio is much greater, causing a higher proportion of head trauma [20]. It is, therefore, essential that pediatric patients be appropriately triaged and evacuated to capable neurotrauma centers. A study looking at blast injury to children during the Oklahoma City bombing showed a high proportion of severe head injury [21], and retrospective studies have shown a difference in injury patterns in children when compared to adults after a blast injury [22].

Management of a child's airways differs significantly from an adult, to the point that even an experienced emergency medical service provider may have difficulty if they are insufficiently trained. A large tongue, poorly anchored teeth, and a compliant trachea all must be taken into consideration when providing treatment [20]. The healthcare provider must know that the most common cause of cardiac arrest in a child is hypoxia, therefore the importance of an established airway cannot be overstressed. Simple details such as proper head positioning may be a lifesaving maneuver by preventing hypoxia. Pediatric expert opinions in disaster scenarios have suggested focusing on correct positioning and bag valve mask ventilation in the pre-hospital setting instead of invasive airways [3]. Yet, devoting a skilled individual to maintaining an airway while "bagging" the child requires additional manpower in a scenario already characterized by a paucity of qualified care providers. The availability of working suction is also a vital step in accessing and maintaining an airway, especially a pediatric airway where the smaller diameter is more easily occluded.

Infants have a greater surface area to body mass and more permeable skin than adults. The skin is less keratinized, leaving it more vulnerable to erosive injury and burn [23]. Both of these factors result in a higher absorption of toxins and a larger surface area to be potentially injured by any kind of trauma (chemical, biological, heat, cold, penetrating, blunt, or blast). For example, even a small percentage of body surface with significant burn injury (an amount which would not be so morbid in an adult) can have detrimental consequences to an infant. Serious burns during an MCI carry a high mortality rate, are difficult for the first-response team to treat, and demand a high level of specific care (preferably a verified burn center).

A child in hemodynamic shock presents significantly differently than their adult counterpart. A child will be able to maintain blood pressure even after significant blood loss and may not present with hypotension until 25–50% of total blood volume has been lost [20]. Difficulty in identifying shock in infants is especially challenging, given their unique symptom presentation which ranges from hyper- or hypo-ventilation, changes in skin rigor, glucose intolerance, or metabolic instability.

The greater respiratory rate of children and infants creates a larger intake of airborne chemicals, biological warfare agents, smoke, and dust secondary to the natural or provoked disaster [24]. This is due to both the higher oxygen consumption of the child per minute, and the child being physically closer to the ground. For example, a 6-month-old child has an average oxygen consumption rate of 7 mL/kg/min compared to a healthy adult average of 3.5 mL/kg/min, effectively doubling the inhalation of any present toxic substances. The proximity to the ground makes a more hazardous "breathing zone" because of the natural gravitational fall of the heavier compounds, such as aerosol gases sarin and chloride and radioactive particles such as radon [25]. The higher baseline heart rate of children then causes the inhaled toxic substance to circulate throughout the child's body more rapidly. These toxins are also metabolized differently than in adults because of certain aspects of a child's/infant's physiology, including a slower GI absorption, higher body water concentration, limited protein binding ability, larger liver-mass-to-body ratio, immature renal function, and a more permeable blood–brain barrier [26]. It is also crucial that the differences in children's metabolism be considered in dosing potential curative or preventive medications/vaccines/antidotes.

The infant/child's larger body water ratio leaves them more vulnerable to the elements during the disorder of an MCI. They are more easily overheated (therefore leading to dehydration), especially when still young enough to be dependent upon being given water. For infants, a bottle, or lactating woman, may not be available. Dehydration can be exacerbated by toxic agents causing diarrhea or vomiting. The electrolyte balances of children are also more vulnerable to change, and their imbalances may easily lead to potentially fatal abnormalities that are difficult to diagnose, especially in an out-of-hospital setting [27]. Breastfeeding, when available, may be the only access to sanitary water and calorie intake for an infant. Studies have shown that, during times of desperate need, the ability to initiate lactation in pregnant women in whom lactation has not begun, or to re-initiate lactation in mothers recently after delivery who are not breastfeeding [20], can save lives. Breastfeeding does, however, rely on the mother receiving adequate nutrition in order to continue producing sufficient milk, which may be an issue during a community-wide disaster.

Children's physical and mental limitations, along with their dependence on adults for survival, also put them at higher risk for injury and death. They lack the physical capability and motor skills to avoid danger and, until a certain age, do not possess the cognitive ability to assess, react to, and escape a dangerous situation. Although these skills may be taught at a relatively young age (for example, preschool age children learning how to dial a specific number for help), it has been shown to take weeks of organized teaching and does not take into account the fear accompanying an acute event [28]. Young children cannot express what they need

Table 12.1 The major anatomical and physiological differences between children and adults

Anatomical differences
– Larger head-to-body ratio
– Larger surface area-to-body mass ratio
– Closure together and less protected internal organs
– Smaller airway, potential loose teeth, compliant trachea
– More permeable and fragile skin
– Closure to the ground
Physiological differences
– Shock presented differently; greater ability to compensate hemorrhagic shock
– Greater respiratory and pulse rate
– Larger water-to-body mass ratio
– Different gastrointestinal absorption and metabolism

or feel, which may exacerbate misdiagnoses and delays in treatment, especially by the provider untrained in pediatrics. In the chaos immediately after the MCI, children still remain at significant danger due to their natural curiosity and vulnerability and have disproportionately been victims of violent and sexual crimes [29].

All MCI include some variation of transport, whether for escape purposes or conveyance to treatment centers. When transporting a child or infant, their physical size must be taken into account in order to avoid preventable accidents. Proper restraints, or even the most basic knowledge on how to correctly apply the restraints, have been shown to be lacking in the day-to-day transport via ambulance of a variety of ages of children [30].

A summary of the major anatomical and physiological differences seen in children is summarized in Table 12.1.

12.2 Treatment

As in any medical setting, be it a military field hospital or state-of-the-art urban hospital, pediatric patients demand certain expertise, training, and equipment during all aspects of care (from transport to definitive procedures). The treatment starts with a knowledge of injury patterns, depending on the cause of the MCI. For example an injury profile from terrorist events in Israel showed that over 70% of the children had head injury, followed by the lower extremities, upper extremities, and body [31].The mechanism of injury must be understood according to the age groups injured, and their specific needs, signs, and symptoms. If biological or chemical warfare is present, the initial approach to a child might be challenging in protective suits which might frighten the child to the point of refusing to allow treatment. Additionally, the small procedures, such as an IV line, will be difficult to accomplish in the bulky clothing and gloves if not previously practiced [32]. Details about biological and chemical pathogens are discussed in greater details in other chapters in this book. The major biological pathogens, chemical agents, and physical injuries for which pre-emptive preparedness is essential are summarized in Table 12.2. Being prepared for any of these mechanisms of injury means being able to rapidly

Table 12.2 A summary of the major potential biological, chemical, and MCI injuries to children

Method of injury	Comments
Biological	
Anthrax	Respiratory or cutaneous symptoms
Plague	
Tularemia	
Smallpox	Vaccine not approved for children less than 12 months
Botulism	
Chemical	
Nerve gases	Examples: Tabun, Sarin, Soman, VX
Vesicants	Examples: Mustard gas, Nitrogen mustard
Choking agents	Examples: Phosgene
Cyanogens	Examples: Hydrogen cyanide
Irritants	Examples: Chlorine, Bromine, Ammonia
Central nervous system depressants	Examples: Cannabinoids, Barbiturates
Physical	Significant injury, most probably a combination of the injuries listed below, need rapid transport to definitive care. Tourniquet application essential when needed
Penetrating injury	
Blast injury	
Crush injury	
Burn injury	

and accurately diagnose, understand signs/symptoms and isolation needs, and have treatments and prophylaxis easily available to administer in the correct pediatric doses.

The use of blood products must also be mentioned, previous studies have shown that up to 1/3 of patients during suicide bombings required blood products which were usually given within the first 2 h of treatment [33]. Access to blood products in the field is more readily available and utilized, nevertheless it is not arbitrary giving blood products to children, and specific volumes must be accurately given. Therefore without pre-emptive protocols, or available expertise, the use of blood products may be dangerously underutilized or utilized in a harmful manner. Within the hospital, the blood bank must be among the first made aware of a MCI and the flux of trauma patients. A standard operation procedure must be in place and activated in order to maintain a pool of blood products and to rapidly and accurately continue to dispense the blood products as needed [18].

12.3 Social Issues

The social issues surrounding children during a MCI cannot be underestimated or ignored. Issues such as reunification and basic comfort are as important as medical care and, if neglected, have the potential to compromise the entire rescue effort through the consumption of excess effort and additional manpower. In order to ensure child safety, any child presenting for care must be assumed to be alone, or "orphaned," until proven otherwise. These children must be cared for and protected throughout mobilization and definitive care until appropriate parents or family members present themselves.

Reunification remains an issue after even the most recent MCI occurring during the era of advanced communication technology and social media. Even for healthy children, significant planning and coordination is required in order to safeguard, transport, and properly reunify the child with their family after the MCI [34]. The temporary caregivers (whether an individual or an organization) suddenly have complete responsibility for reunifying the child in a safe environment with their true family. Certain methods theoretically and practically exist to assist with children after an MCI, including secure tracking systems with personal information to be utilized only during an emergency situation, education for healthcare workers on proper identification to ensure safe and correct reunification, and "pediatric safe" shelters for children waiting to be reunified. However, these programs must be pre-emptively organized, practiced, and prepared for, and will most likely be lacking in organization during the initial phase of the MCI. To help in decreasing the potential amount of chaos, there must be an area designated for "parent information" in a location away from triage that will not hinder patient care, will help with reunification, and try to answer parents' questions and decrease their concerns.

The correlation between a traumatic event in childhood (or even while in-utero) and negative effects to health and quality of life as an adult has been established [35, 36]. Post-traumatic stress disorder after certain MCI has affected the majority of children involved, both healthy and injured, with symptoms lasting for an extended duration [37]. Therefore, the social support for children, whether casualties or not, indirectly or directly affected by the MCI must be handled in the acute setting with the highest level of importance and care.

Conclusion

As disasters continue to occur, the lack of preparedness and deficiencies when dealing with the pediatric population continue to be documented and fatally affect the care of children. These deficiencies have motivated the medical and emergency service communities to increase the amount and level of training for a "surge" of pediatric patients. Technological advancements have also aided in communities being better prepared for MCI involving children. One example of enhanced hospital preparedness is the use of geographic information systems (GIS) to accurately predict potential pediatric "surges" during a disaster [38], thereby enabling a hospital to be better prepared in terms of manpower (pediatric specialists), pediatric supplies, and appropriate medicine doses. Due to the variety of MCI and the immense differences between locations where MCI occur (urban vs. rural, poor vs. rich community), adequate preparation is extremely difficult even under optimal conditions. Nevertheless, understanding the specific needs of the pediatric population is the first step in delivering optimal care under extreme circumstances.

Certain points that must be stressed:

1. "Children are not small adults" (a wise pediatrician once said), in regard to physiology, anatomy, medications, and supportive needs. This is relevant starting from the first encounter with a pediatric victim, from triage to definitive care.
2. Pediatricians/pediatric surgeons/pediatric emergency and intensivist physicians need to be involved in every step of a community's MCI preparation, protocol creation, and deployment. First-response teams, non-pediatric emergency rooms, and any potential triaging officer or professional giving medical or logistical care to children must consistently train with pediatric scenarios and equipment. Leaders from the local school district may also play an important role in these preparations. Large and small scale drills must occur routinely.
3. A significant and crucial role for volunteers (an influx sometimes sufficient to overwhelm and hinder the rescue operation) can be functioning as parental figures/caretakers for orphaned or displaced children during all stages of the process (triage, treatment, transport, hospitalization/definitive care) until the reunification process is complete. This would remove a significant burden from the healthcare and rescue workers, allowing them to utilize their training more efficiently. Obviously, safety issues must be acknowledged and considered, but there might not be a choice during a time of chaos and desperation.
4. Treatment facilities—whether originating from the backpack of a military medic, ambulance, field hospital, or definitive care hospital—must be prepared with the practical supplies in the appropriate sizes for pediatric patients. This includes: child/family friendly decontamination facilities, airways, chest tubes, and pediatric dosages of medicines/antidotes. An area designated for pediatrics will help decrease confusion and smooth diagnosis, treatments, and transport.
5. Acknowledge and act to prevent potential "secondary injuries" to the children. This includes everything that is not a physical injury—from decreasing the stress of the child (i.e., by early reunification), to keeping them safe.

Acknowledgment *Thank you to Krystin Johnson, of Austin, Texas, for her editorial expertise.*

References

1. http://data.worldbank.org/indicator/SP.POP.0014.TO.ZS.
2. Seidel JS, Hornbein M, Yoshiyama K, Kuznets D, Finklestein JZ, St Geme JW. Emergency medical services and the pediatric patient: are the needs being met? Pediatrics. 1984;73(6):769–72.
3. Lyle K, Thompson T, Graham J. Pediatric mass casualty: triage and planning for the prehospital provider. Clin Pediatr Emerg Med. 2009;10(3):173–85.
4. Gausche-Hill M, Schmitz C, Lewis RJ. Pediatric preparedness of US emergency departments: a 2003 survey. Pediatrics. 2007;120(6):1229–37.
5. Chung S, Shannon M. Hospital planning for acts of terrorism and other public health emergencies involving children. Arch Dis Childhood. 2005;90(12):1300–7.

6. Ferrer RR, Ramirez M, Sauser K, Iverson E, Upperman JS. Emergency drills and exercises in healthcare organizations: assessment of pediatric population involvement using after-action reports. Am J Disaster Med. 2008;4(1):23–32.
7. Shirm S, Liggin R, Dick R, Graham J. Prehospital preparedness for pediatric mass-casualty events. Pediatrics. 2007;120(4):e756–61.
8. Markenson D, Redlener I. Pediatric terrorism preparedness national guidelines and recommendations: findings of an evidenced-based consensus process. Biosecur Bioterror. 2004;2(4):301–19.
9. Manoj BS, Baker AH. Communication challenges in emergency response. Commun ACM. 2007;50(3):51–3.
10. Lerner EB, Schwartz RB, Coule PL, Weinstein ES, Cone DC, Hunt RC, Sasser SM, Liu JM, Nudell NG, Wedmore IS, Hammond J. Mass casualty triage: an evaluation of the data and development of a proposed national guideline. Disaster Med Public Health Prep. 2008;2(S1):S25–34.
11. Jones N, White ML, Tofil N, Pickens M, Youngblood A, Zinkan L, Baker MD. Randomized trial comparing two mass casualty triage systems (JumpSTART versus SALT) in a pediatric simulated mass casualty event. Prehosp Emerg Care. 2014;18(3):417–23.
12. Waisman Y, Amir L, Mor M, Feigenberg Z, Aharonson LD, Peleg K, Blumenfeld A. Prehospital response and field triage in pediatric mass casualty incidents: the Israeli experience. Clin Pediatr Emerg Med. 2006;7(1):52–8.
13. Wallis LA, Carley S. Comparison of paediatric major incident primary triage tools. Emerg Med J. 2006;23(6):475–8.
14. Nadeau NL, Cicero MX. Pediatric disaster triage system utilization across the United States. Pediatr Emerg Care. 2017;33(3):152–5.
15. Ma OJ, Norvell JG, Subramanian S. Ultrasound applications in mass casualties and extreme environments. Crit Care Med. 2007;35(5):S275–9.
16. Ong AW, McKenney MG, McKenney KA, Brown M, Namias N, MaCloud J, Cohn SM. Predicting the need for laparotomy in pediatric trauma patients on the basis of the ultrasound score. J Trauma Acute Care Surg. 2003;54(3):503–8.
17. Barthel ER, Pierce JR, Goodhue CJ, Burke RV, Ford HR, Upperman JS. Can a pediatric trauma center improve the response to a mass casualty incident? J Trauma Acute Care Surg. 2012;73(4):885–9.
18. Soffer D, Klausner JM. Trauma system configurations in other countries: the Israeli model. Surg Clin North Am. 2012;92(4):1025–40.
19. Burke RV, Iverson E, Goodhue CJ, Neches R, Upperman JS. Disaster and mass casualty events in the pediatric population. Semin Pediatr Surg. 2010;19(4):265–70. WB Saunders.
20. Kissoon N, Dreyer J, Walia M. Pediatric trauma: differences in pathophysiology, injury patterns and treatment compared with adult trauma. CMAJ. 1990;142(1):27.
21. Quintana DA, Jordan FB, Tuggle DW, Mantor PC, Tunell WP. The spectrum of pediatric injuries after a bomb blast. J Pediatr Surg. 1997;32(2):307–11.
22. Goldstein AL, Klausner JM, Soffer D. Not a blunt issue, but penetrating-an Israeli experience with abdominal injury in civilian multiple casualty blast incidents. Am Surg. 2014;80(1):98.
23. Markenson D, Reynolds S. The pediatrician and disaster preparedness. Pediatrics. 2006;117(2):e340–62.
24. Committee on Environmental Health, Committee on Infectious Diseases. Chemical-biological terrorism and its impact on children: a subject review. Pediatrics. 2000;105(3):662–70.
25. Bearer CF. How are children different from adults? Environ Health Perspect. 1995;103(Suppl 6):7.
26. Stephenson T. How children's responses to drugs differ from adults. Br J Clin Pharmacol. 2005;59(6):670–3.
27. Chilton LA. Prevention and management of hypernatremic dehydration in breast-fed infants. West J Med. 1995;163(1):74.
28. Jones RT. Teaching children to make emergency telephone calls. J Black Psychol. 1980;6(2):81–93.

29. Garrett AL, Grant R, Madrid P, Brito A, Abramson D, Redlener I. Children and megadisasters: lessons learned in the new millennium. Adv Pediatr. 2007;54(1):189–214.
30. Johnson TD, Lindholm D, Dowd MD. Child and provider restraints in ambulances: knowledge, opinions, and behaviors of emergency medical services providers. Acad Emerg Med. 2006;13(8):886–92.
31. Waisman Y, Aharonson-Daniel L, Mor M, Amir L, Peleg K. The impact of terrorism on children: a two-year experience. Prehosp Disaster Med. 2003;18(3):242–8.
32. Redlener I, Markenson D. Disaster and terrorism preparedness: what pediatricians need to know. Dis Mon. 2004;50(1):6–40.
33. Bala M, Kaufman T, Keidar A, Zelig O, Zamir G, Mudhi-Orenshat S, Bdolah-Abram T, Rivkind AI, Almogy G. Defining the need for blood and blood products transfusion following suicide bombing attacks on a civilian population: a level I single-centre experience. Injury. 2014;45(1):50–5.
34. Blake N, Stevenson K. Reunification: keeping families together in crisis. J Trauma Acute Care Surg. 2009;67(2):S147–51.
35. King S, Dancause K, Turcotte-Tremblay AM, Veru F, Laplante DP. Using natural disasters to study the effects of prenatal maternal stress on child health and development. Birth Defects Res C Embryo Today. 2012;96(4):273–88.
36. Almond D, Currie J. Killing me softly: the fetal origins hypothesis. J Econ Perspect. 2011;25(3):153–72.
37. Pynoos RS, Goenjian A, Tashjian M, Karakashian M, Manjikian R, Manoukian G, Steinberg AM, Fairbanks LA. Post-traumatic stress reactions in children after the 1988 Armenian earthquake. Br J Psychiatry. 1993;163(2):239–47.
38. Curtis JW, Curtis A, Upperman JS. Using a geographic information system (GIS) to assess pediatric surge potential after an earthquake. Disaster Med Public Health Prep. 2012;6(2):163–9.

Definitive Care Phase of a Mass Casualty Incident

13

Offir Ben-Ishay

13.1 Introduction

Mass Casualty Incident (MCI) is an event that overwhelm the local healthcare system with a number of casualties that vastly exceed the local resources and capabilities in a short period of time. This definition puts an emphasis on the local resources of a particular hospital, as the affirmation of an ongoing MCI is different from one hospital to another, meaning that an MCI for one hospital is only a relatively busy day for another.

A mass casualty incident can be divided into three phases [1–5] as follows:

- *Phase 1*—Starts when the incident is reported and the level of response is defined. Central command sets the number of ambulances needed, the number of EMS districts that should be activated, and the number of hospitals that should activate their MCI protocols. The hospitals on their end being aware of their surge capacity should create extra capacity in the hospital starting in the Emergency Department by discharging patients who are amendable for discharge and admitting the ones who are not. Extra capacity should also be created on the floors by cancelling elective cases and patients awaiting discharge should be readily discharged.
- *Phase 2*—During the second phase, evacuation of the critical (immediate) patients from the scene begins, followed by the serious (urgent) patients. These patients are treated with the confined area of the immediate patients (trauma shock room) or in the emergency department itself. Minor patients (delayed) that

O Ben-Ishay (✉)
Surgical Oncology, Department of General Surgery,
Rambam Health Care Campus, Haifa, Israel
e-mail: o_ben-ishay@rambam.health.gov.il

Y. Kluger et al. (eds.), *WSES Handbook of Mass Casualties Incidents Management*, Hot Topics in Acute Care Surgery and Trauma,
https://doi.org/10.1007/978-3-319-92345-1_13

were evacuated from the scene or arrived to the hospital independently are treated with the concept of minimal acceptable care.

- Phase 2 should end within the first 6 h. Although no prospective randomized trial exists regarding, studies show though, that the quality of care steeply decreases 6–8 h from the onset of the event, due to team exhaustion.
- *Phase 3*—Is the delayed care phase; this is the time to treat the minor injuries (delayed patients), perform a tertiary survey, take care of the secondary distribution of patients and debrief the team.

13.2 The Concept Minimal Acceptable Care

When MCI patients arrive to the Emergency Department (ED) in waves, the first wave consists of patients that are able to walk and do not need any type of evacuation or extrication. These patients will arrive to the hospital in the first 15–30 min and their time of arrival really depends on the distance of the hospital from the scene. The effect of the first wave is well noticed within the first few minutes as they crowd the ED creating initial unjustified chaos and they should be triaged and directed towards the delayed patients' pre-designated area prior to the arrival of the second wave [6].

The second wave of patients includes those who require EMS transport and may include those in urgent need of immediate care. These patients should also be triaged and be treated accordingly.

The third wave consists of the patients that need long extrication time, and often these patients have combined injuries composed of penetrating, blunt, blast, and secondary hits attributed to hypovolaemia and crash injuries.

In the past, patients in the second and third phase were treated with the concept of "the greater good for the greater number of patients" in terms of doing your best for the largest number of patients, taking into consideration some compromise in the quality of care given. Currently, this concept is no longer acceptable and we should give the same high level of care to a critically injured patient during an MCI as it was an everyday care. This concept requires excellent field triage and patient's distribution, and even better hospital triage.

Retrospective analysis of past MCIs shows that only 10% of the victims are in need of life-saving procedures and are severely injured, most of the patients have minor or stress-related injuries. The concept of minimal acceptable care was developed in order to treat those minor injuries for the best at first and delay the definitive care for later. This concept allows the trauma teams to allocate the necessary resources to the severely injured allowing them to give high level of care for those in real need and offload the trauma service line and other bottlenecks such as CT scan and the operating theatre.

Examples of minimal acceptable care are patients with simple long bone fractures that will be treated with simple splint or cast before getting a definitive treatment and complete operative reduction and fixation. In extremis even hemodynamic stable patient with penetrating injury to the abdomen, who is in obvious need of exploratory laparotomy, may be delayed in the surgical floor or the ICU for definitive surgical treatment during the delayed care phase.

13.3 Definitive Care Phase

13.3.1 Treatment for Minor Injuries

When all is set and done, and all patients were evacuated from the scene, the definite number of injured is known and the severely injured are appropriately treated and allocated in the ICU or in the surgical floors; it is time to treat the minor injuries. These patients were displaced after proper triage to a pre-designated area for the delayed patients. The medical and paramedical teams, which are allocated in this area, are support teams from other departments in the hospital and are not used to treat trauma patients. Therefore once the trauma teams have the necessary time and resources a *secondary survey* should be deployed and patients with minor injuries should be re-examined and treated accordingly. Those in need of further imaging and treatment should be treated accordingly and those amendable for discharge should be discharged as soon as possible.

13.3.2 Tertiary Survey

Once the number of injured patients is known and their bed allocation is well described; a thorough-doctors grand rounds should take place. Each patient should go through a repeat and complete history and physical examination and the extent of his injuries and treatment received so far should be re-evaluated.

The main goal of this survey is to reduce to the minimum the incidence of missed injuries and to obtain a list of prioritized needs of patients for imaging, operative procedures, or other limited resources. The tertiary survey will determine the need to transfer of patients to other medical facilities for specialized care or reduction of waiting times for definitive operative treatment or reduction of workload of the already exhausted teams.

13.4 Secondary Distribution

Patient's distribution starts from the concept of field triage, Patients are divided to Critical (immediate), Serious (urgent) and minor (delayed) injuries. Furthermre, EMS should be aware of the level of care provided in each hospital and should distribute the patients accordingly. Furthermore, EMS should be aware of the subspecialties that exist in each hospital and should distribute the patients accordingly.

Many concerns exist regarding the treatment capabilities of each hospital, and this should be well-defined, pre-planned, and well-practiced. Unfortunately, often the surge capacity of hospitals is outdated and based on an irrelevant number of hospital beds.

Patient's distribution protocols are in place to allow hospitals not to go over their maximum capacity by allocating casualties to several hospitals, equally distributing not only the severe injuries but also the minor ones. Conflicts occure when hopsitals and EMS do not share the same distribution protocols and if they the actually do, the EMS staff is not aware of them or within the mayhem created during an MCI protocols are disrigarded [7–9].

Failed secondary distribution of patients could occur due to:

- Wrongful triage (in field, in transport, in hospital and secondary triage) and this should be reduced to the minimum.
- Need for specialized care—assuming that the triage was correct, this is unexpected, it requires transport services of the EMS and significant medical, paramedical, and administrative resources that add up to the already immense burden of care.
- Re-distribution of the burden of the definitive care. This is expected but still requires significant resources that are not always available.

13.4.1 Debriefing

A formal debriefing of all the staff that took part in the joint effort of treating the MCI is a crucial final step. The debriefing should be structured and should cover all the medical, paramedical, and administrative areas that are relevant. Each member of the staff should be able to speak freely of his experience and all points should be taken into consideration.

The goal of debriefing is to teach the necessary lessons and improve the hospital response plan for an MCI.

In conclusion, the definitive care phase is a crucial component of an MCI management and it takes a considerable amount of time and resources; it should be inserted into the hospital MCI protocol and practised routinely. Although the ED may return to normal activity fairly quickly, in the ICU and the OR, this may take days to weeks.

References

1. Aylwin CJ, Konig TC, Brennan NW, et al. Reduction in critical mortality in urban mass casualty incidents: analysis of triage, surge, and resource use after the London bombings on July 7, 2005. Lancet. 2006;368:2219–25.
2. Cushman JG, Pachter HL, Beaton HL. Two New York City hospitals' surgical response to the September 11, 2001, terrorist attack in New York City. J Trauma. 2003;54:147–54.
3. Frykberg ER. Medical management of disasters and mass casualties from terrorist bombings: how can we cope? J Trauma. 2002;53:201–12.

4. Stein M, Hirshberg A. Medical consequences of terrorism. The conventional weapon threat. Surg Clin North Am. 1999;79:1537–52.
5. Einav S, Aharonson-Daniel L, Weissman C, et al. In-hospital resource utilization during multiple casualty incidents. Ann Surg. 2006;243:533–40.
6. Coupland RM. Epidemiological approach to surgical management of the casualties of war. BMJ. 1994;308:1693–7.
7. Aschkenasy-Steuer G, Shamir M, Rivkind A, et al. Clinical review: the Israeli experience: conventional terrorism and critical care. Crit Care. 2005;9:490–9.
8. Ozoilo KN, Pam IC, Yiltok SJ, et al. Challenges of the management of mass casualty: lessons learned from the Jos crisis of 2001. World J Emerg Surg. 2013;8:44.
9. Hirshberg A, Scott BG, Granchi T, et al. How does casualty load affect trauma care in urban bombing incidents? A quantitative analysis. J Trauma. 2005;58:686–93.

Preparedness to Non-conventional Incidents in the Civilian Medical Arena

14

G. Shaked, D. Czeiger, and G. Sebbag

14.1 Background

There is no doubt that for many years the threat of weapons of mass destruction (WMD) imposes a great concern on citizens as well as on nation leaders. President Bush recognized the possibility of a secret and sudden attack with chemical or nuclear weapons as the greatest threat before humanity [1]. Since the first use of chemical agents in modern era during World War I, very few examples were documented where non-conventional weapon (NCW) was used by a state. However, in the Middle-East region in recent years several chemical attacks have been carried out in Syria by the government forces against their opponents, and in the 1980s by Iraq forces against Kurd civilians. The response of the international community against these incidents was much more significant than the one given after conventional attacks that caused a higher death toll along the years of fighting. This reflects the fear and different attitude that people and governments have towards the use of NCW. The September 11, 2001 terror attack in New York was the turning point of modern terrorism. The large number of casualties, the serious economic damage, and the psychological effects of this "mega-terrorism event" were unprecedented. It was expected that this achievement of a single terror attack would encourage terror groups to mimic it by attempting more conventional mega-terrorism attacks, or using non-conventional materials that would cause the same effect [2]. Although seemingly NCW can be considered an ideal choice for terrorist organizations, only very few terrorist attacks using these materials have been carried out in the past [3]. Non-conventional mass-casualty events (MCE) may be caused by toxicological, radiation, or biological agent dissemination. The MCE may be of natural cause, like a global viral flu event (e.g., the Spanish flu in 1918–1920 with millions of deaths) or a MCE

G. Shaked (✉) · D. Czeiger · G. Sebbag
Department of General Surgery, Soroka University Medical Center and Ben-Gurion University, Beer Sheva, Israel

Y. Kluger et al. (eds.), *WSES Handbook of Mass Casualties Incidents Management*, Hot Topics in Acute Care Surgery and Trauma,
https://doi.org/10.1007/978-3-319-92345-1_14

after a terrorism act like the Anthrax envelope scare in Boca Raton, Florida in 2001. Best known chemical incidents in a civilian setup are the attacks carried out in Japan by the Aum Shinrikyo (Supreme Trust) group in 1994–1995. In the Tokyo subway attack in 1995 which involved releasing sarin nerve gas, twelve were killed and thousands injured. In 2007, multiple terrorist bombings had been reported in Iraq using chlorine gas. Recently in 2018, a former Russian spy and his daughter were supposedly poisoned in London by a potent nerve gas. Toxicological incidents can occur not just by a terrorist act but also and even more often as an accident, for example an explosion in a chemical factory producing hazardous materials, or a road accident of a truck transferring such materials. Radiological materials can find their way to terrorist organizations that might use them to make a "dirty bomb." This low-tech radiological weapon is actually a conventional explosive bomb with a radiation side effect. Although the radiation effect will probably be negligible compared to a nuclear bomb, it can induce a heavy emotional impact and neutralize large contaminated areas. Until now, only few terrorist attacks using radiation materials have been reported. In 1995 and 1998, two attempts of dirty bombs use by a Chechen group were thwarted. Another case is the radiation poisoning of Alexander Litvinenko, a former KGB agent, by ingestion of Polonium∗210. A radiation event may also be the result of an accident in a nuclear plant, in a medical isotopes imaging institution, or in a laboratory using radiation materials. In all the forms of non-conventional events, the victims may suffer from the combination of conventional and non-conventional injuries, or either one of these types of injury. Bio-terrorism is even rarer though it is also very tempting to terrorists to use. Different US security organizations as well as other governments share a global war against terror. That includes the fight to prevent the possible use of NCW by terror organizations. The efforts and resources are aimed on the four premises of deterrence, prevention, defense, and consequence management [4]. The fact that the incidental use of NCW is relatively so scarce is encouraging and emphasizes the vital continuous need for international supervision of the development, manufacture, and marketing of NCW, and for coordinated steps to prevent access by unauthorized groups to these agents. Unfortunately, there is always a chance that the ability and the motivation of a terrorist group will meet and will result in translating the potential into reality. The probability of such an event has even increased in the last decade after the disintegration of states like Libya, Iraq, and Syria that made their military NCW arsenal easily available to different terror organizations. In most if not all NCW attacks, the nation health system is almost immediately involved. As a consequence of the described situation, the civilian health system must be prepared to non-conventional incidents. This chapter delineates the challenges, preparedness, special equipment, and organizational requirements that a medical center faces when dealing with a non-conventional MCE.

14.2 General Considerations

Terrorist act or an accident in an industrialized area may result in combined conventional and non-conventional injuries that may affect tens to thousands of people if it happens in a heavily populated area. The number of victims and the severity of their injuries depend on the population density, the type of agent, its quantity, its toxicity, and the meteorological conditions at the time of incident. Explosion and fire aggravate the agent effects, making the rescue efforts more complicated. Non-conventional incidents are fortunately rare but this fact just strengthen the need for awareness of health systems to such possibility and to prepare to it, and it requires the awareness of the medical teams in order to promptly identify an event once it occurs and to modify the management accordingly. As is true to all types of MCE, timely and rapid organization of the emergency medical services (EMS) and medical centers is crucial for an efficient and successful response. Medical centers should map and evaluate the risks of non-conventional event in their area. For example, the presence of a nuclear plant, medical or university laboratories using radiation compounds, traffic of trucks or trains loaded with hazardous materials, concrete threat of terrorism, etc. It is important to appoint a team to be in charge of organizing the standard operating procedures (SOP) protocols for each type of MCE, to assimilate and implement the knowledge and guidelines among the medical, paramedical, logistic, and assisting teams, and on keeping the preparedness of the hospital by performing periodical drills. It is important to remember that although it is recommended to follow the basic principles of MCE any single medical center needs to prepare its own SOP and the way it organizes and controls the situation by making the local necessary adaptations. Variables like the topography of the admitting area, available personnel in different daily times, size of the treatment area, capacity of the hospital, number of victims that can be managed in a single wave, mechanical ventilators availability, capacity of blood bank, availability of surgical rooms, intensive care beds, options for secondary evacuation of patients to other facilities, and so on may affect the way a certain hospital will establish its plan. The accepted evaluation in Israel is that the admitting surge capability of a hospital in a single wave of victims of MCE should be 20% of the total hospital beds during regular activity. The working assumption is that the admitting hospital itself is not contaminated. However, there are two scenarios for the initial management of non-conventional event. An "overt exposure situation" when it is clear from the pre-hospital phase that the injured are also contaminated by a toxic or radiological substance, as opposed to an "unknown exposure situation" when the fact of contamination is not initially identified. In the second scenario, patients enter the emergency department normally and contaminate the entire area and those who come in contact with them. Clear separation marked by a colored line on the floor should be made to sign the border between "dirty" and "clean" areas. The victims should be evacuated from the contaminated scene as fast as possible. Lifesaving procedures, undressing, cleansing, and treatment with antidote (if appropriate) will be done en route. Resources should not be expended on patients who have experienced a cardiac or respiratory arrest if there are large numbers of casualties requiring care above the capabilities of the health providers. Special care is given to health providers' safety. Once a definite diagnosis has been made that a hazardous material is involved, special precautions should be followed including wearing specific protective gear for team members who come in contact with contaminated victims. It should be remembered that communication between team members that wear protective gear including gas masks and between this team and the person who controls the event may be problematic. Another special issue in coping with non-conventional event is that it is expected that a large number of healthy worried citizens and people suffering from acute stress reaction would flood the health system.

14.3 Toxicological/Chemical Event

EMS transfer casualties to the hospital, usually after the first decontamination process if available. This process at the scene is appropriate only in stable patients. Patients sustaining immediate life-threatening condition will be entered into a resuscitation bay without decontamination. A resuscitation area is allocated adjacent to the ambulance unloading point, or, as it is the case in our medical center, in a pre-designed "dirty" area inside the shock-trauma room. In such a case that part of the room becomes contaminated and is separated from the other bays. The team in the "dirty" area works wearing protective gear. Following the initial resuscitation, wet cleansing is performed and the patient will be transferred across to the "clean" areas of the emergency room for further treatment. The diagnosis and identification of involvement of toxic material can be based on early information from the scene or based on the clinical presentation of the first arriving patients. Upon the recognition of a toxic material an immediate contact is made with the toxicology expert, if there is one in the hospital, or with a National Toxicology Center to get more information about the hazardous material, its toxicity, special risks and the need for special protective gear, and the availability of an antidote. Another source of information (in Israel) may be the IDF Medical Corps and/or the Home-front Command. Updated contact routes to these agents must be available in the folder for this type of event. Since it is possible that a large number of patients will arrive prior to making the diagnosis of a toxic event, the entire emergency room could become contaminated. It is advisable to prepare for such situations a secondary remote area that will be able to serve for treating later on patients who underwent cleansing. All patients arriving to the hospital must be undressed prior to entering the emergency department. Undressing reduces the exposure to the toxic material by 90%. All contaminated clothes should be collected in HAZMAT plastic bags. After underdressing, the injured undergo wet cleansing. This is done in designated pre-installed external showers. Lying patients will be cleansed on fenestrated gurneys that allow drainage of the contaminated fluids. The body is washed out for 2–4 min and the eyes are flushed with water for 5 min. In a case that the treating team members complain on symptoms suggestive an exposure to toxic material, they should be managed like any other victim. Dry decontamination with absorbent materials as Fuller's earth powder is indicated in cases of non-vaporizing phospho-organics or mustard gas. Wet decontamination will follow the dry (Figs. 14.1 and 14.2). Treatment with the appropriate antidote is given to all victims with symptoms. It is recommended to have a stockpile of automatic injectors of atropine and toxogonin in the emergency supplies of the hospital for phospho-organic compound events. Traumatic injuries should be treated as usual after completing the decontamination process.

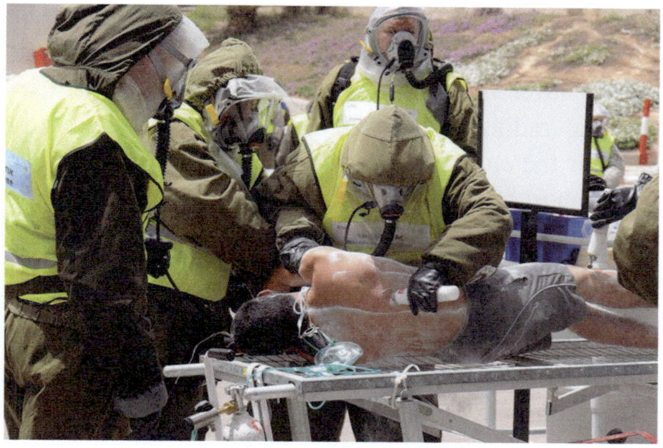

Fig. 14.1 Dry decontamination of a chemical material victim. A drill at Soroka University Medical Center

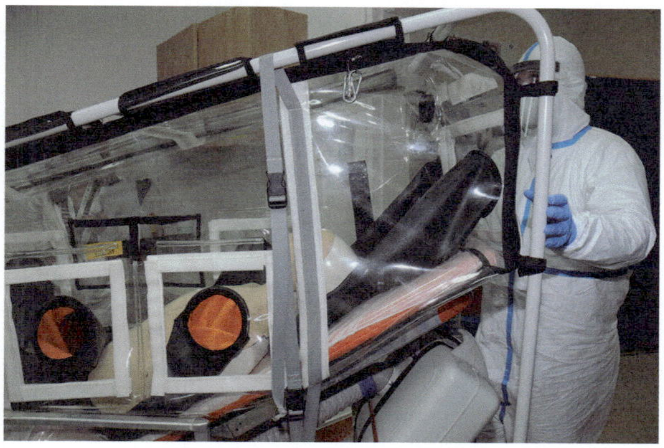

Fig. 14.2 A paramedical staff personnel with bioprotective gear transferring a "patient" in an isolation chamber. A drill at Soroka University Medical Center

14.4 Radiation Event

The management is based on the protocols of a regular MCE with special emphasis on the unique characteristics of this scenario including monitoring and protection of health providers, and the monitoring, decontamination, and treatment of the victims. The management of patients who have been exposed to radiation should preferably be in designated centers with capabilities to provide complicated treatment for radiation burns, internal contamination, or for serious hematological outcome of the sub-acute phase of severe exposure including bone marrow transplantation. Resembling chemical event, radiological event may be "overt" or "unknown." Due to the possibility of a dirty bomb it is now the instruction in Israel and the routine protocol at the Soroka Medical Center to monitor with hand-held radiation detectors every first 3–5 patients who arrive in MCE, to rule out the exposure to radioactive materials. The detectors are posted at the station of the triage nurse and nurses are trained to use them. The psychological effects of a radiation event are extreme and it is expected to receive an unusually large number of worried people and patients with acute stress reactions, so the medical center must be ready with supplementary teams of psychologists and social workers to support these patients. The victims might suffer from several types of damage which include conventional injuries, external radiation, internal radiation, and combined injuries. External radiation exposes the entire body or parts of it to ionizing radiation. The risks for the victim in the short term include acute radiation disease in cases of whole body exposure, and radiation burns in local exposures. The risks in the long term include increased risk for malignancy, harms to offspring, and tissue damage along the tract of the radiation. In these situations, there is no risk to the environment remote from the site of exposure or to the treating teams. In such situations there is no need for decontamination of the patients or to protect the team with special gear. External radioactive contamination is caused by the presence of radioactive material on the body. It may be contaminated liquid, powder, or shell fragments. The risk for the victim is to absorb the external contamination into the body through the respiratory system, the gastrointestinal tract, or through damaged skin. It can also cause local continuous injury to the skin. There is a mild to moderate risk to contaminate the environment and the team although the medical risk for the health providers is low. As a result, it is required to undress the patients as it reduces 90% of the contamination. The undressing should be done gently and the contaminated clothing sealed off in HAZMAT bags. The decontamination process must be also gentle to prevent sprinkling of water on other people and the contaminated water is collected in large plastic bags to prevent further environmental contamination. Team members that act in the "dirty" section at the admitting area including a triage physician, radiation controllers, and nurses that undress and decontaminate the patients should wear protective gear first. Teams that work in the "dirty" bays of the shock-trauma room where they manage the emergent cases that did not undergo initially undressing are also wearing protective gear. Team members who work in the contaminated areas should wear radiation dosimeters. Lifesaving procedures like intubation, decompression of a tension pneumothorax, or control of major bleeding are in priority to decontamination. The contaminated zone floor is covered by special PVC sheaths and these zones are separated from the clean areas by a colored line. It is strictly forbidden for personnel to cross the line. Once the management of a contaminated patient is completed and the patient is now clean, he is transferred from the team in the "dirty" area to another team in the clean zone. Internal contamination happens when radiating material enters the body through the respiratory system, the gastrointestinal tract, or damaged skin. The material is then partly accumulated and partly secreted from the body. The risk to the victim is to develop malignancies, damage to offspring, and rarely severe destruction of target organs. The risk to the team is very low and especially results from direct contact with contaminated secretions. The risk to environment is very low due to dilution of the victim's secretions. Nevertheless, in the acute phase the assumption is that there is also an external contamination so it is required to wear protective gear and to decontaminate the victims. In later phases of the management, it is recommended to collect secretions in order to prevent potential environmental contamination, and to attempt to quantify the internal radioactive load. Using specific antidotes should be considered. In the past years, scientists have been seeking and testing new potential molecules that could be used to decorporate radionuclides in order to treat an internal contamination involving one or several radionuclides [5]. Patients and personnel that attend a radiation incident should receive Lugol iodine pills. Specific medical treatment for internal radioactive contamination may not be available routinely in most hospitals and it is part of the national preparedness to supply these agents to the medical centers that deal with a radiation event. In cases of combined conventional and radiation injuries, the patients should be treated as in regular trauma situations after the decontamination of the patients. The surgical management of radioactive shrapnel requires special attention. The radiation controllers measure the amount of radiation and give directives to the surgical team about safe distance from the agent and safe exposure time, for eventual team replacement. If radiation dose is not excessive, a lead apron and a set of double gloves is enough to protect the surgeon. Contaminated fragments are collected in special vials as all other radioactive materials for disposal.

14.5 Biological Event

This chapter refers only to a biological event that is generated by human usually as a terror act. A biological attack can cause severe mortality, morbidity, disability, impairment of normal life, and anxiety. The incident may progress into a prolonged crisis. The systematic response should aim at lifesaving, prevention of progressive spreading of the causative agent, and minimization of the effects on the routine life of the entire population. The significance of a biological event is far away from the medical center where it was identified. It becomes actually a national and even an international problem. In a case that the event is overt, for example a suspected envelope had been opened in a crowded office; the admitting team should be protected. Rapid identification of the causative agent is very important because the next steps of the management are dependent on it. Anthrax which is considered as one of the preferred infectious agents for biological warfare does not require the isolation of patients. Other diseases may require much complicated management including isolation of patients in special sections, negative pressure rooms, and transferring patients in specified chambers that provide total isolation (Fig. 14.3). Attempt must be made in order to identify all carriers and sick people as early as possible. These efforts are far beyond the medical center itself. Hospital SOP in a biological event is derived according to the magnitude of the event. In a limited event, the identification of contaminated patients is based on high suspicion of the nurses and physicians in the emergency room based on the symptoms and findings of patients. The suspected individuals are isolated in dedicated area (bio-event room) in the emergency room, the health providers who come in contact with the patients must wear protective gear, and all blood and other human secretions are sent to laboratory tests

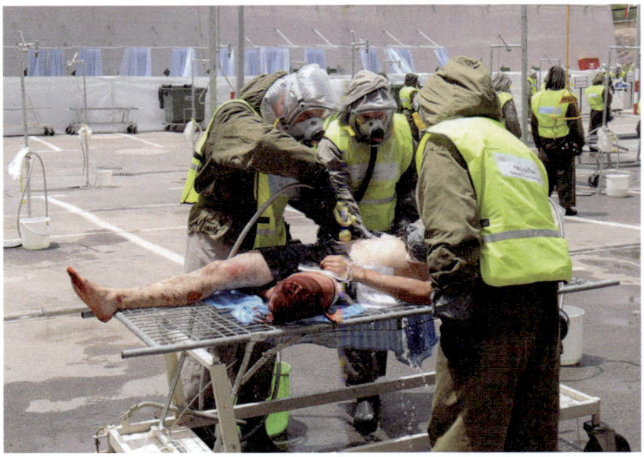

Fig. 14.3 Wet decontamination of a chemical material victim. A drill at Soroka University Medical Center

in biohazard plastic bags. Empiric treatment is started immediately and should be switched to targeted treatment as soon as the definitive diagnosis is made. The institutional infectious disease experts should be promptly involved in the management of the event, and the ministry of health should be informed. The victims are hospitalized in dedicated isolation rooms. In cases of MCE, the entire emergency room is transformed into a "bio emergency room" considering all sections are contaminated. In addition, due to the large numbers of victims a department or even several departments are designated as epidemic hospitalization ward(s).

References

1. President Bush outlines Iraqi threat. October 2002. https://georgewbush-whitehouse.archives.gov/news/releases/2002/10/20021007-8.html.
2. Schweitzer Y. The age on non-conventional terrorism. Strateg Assess. 2003;6(1):26–31. http://www.inss.org.il/publication/the-age-of-non-conventional-terrorism/.
3. Kurz A. Non-conventional terrorism: availability and motivation. Strateg Assess. 2005;7(4):29–35. http://www.inss.org.il/publication/non-conventional-terrorism-availability-and-motivation/.
4. Moodie M. Reducing the biological threat: new thinking, new approaches. Special report 5. Washington: Chemical Biological Arms Control Institute (CBACI); 2003.
5. Steliou K, Faller DV, Pinkert CA, Irwin MH, Moos WH. Bioprotective carnitinoids: lipoic acid, butyrate, and mitochondria-targeting to treat radiation injury: mitochondrial drugs come of age. Drug Dev Res. 2015;76(4):167–75. https://doi.org/10.1002/ddr.21258.

Mass Casualties Management in Low-Income Countries

15

Paola Fugazzola, Federico Coccolini, Cecilia Merli, Emiliano Gamberini, Vanni Agnoletti, and Luca Ansaloni

15.1 Disasters in Low-Income Countries

The terms *disaster* and *mass casualty incident* (MCI) are often used as synonyms, but they describe different entities in terms of discrepancy between the number of victims and the treatment capacity of the community [1]. In MCI, the number of casualties may strain the responding facilities, but resources are sufficient to cope without outside support. A disaster is a catastrophic event which disrupts the social and community infrastructures and extraordinary means are necessary to cope it, resulting in the need for support from the outside [1].

Average mortality for all types of natural disasters increased to 69,800 per years in the decade 2006–2015, up from 64,900 between 1996 and 2005. Average deaths per disaster also rose, up to 194 from 187. These increases reflect the impacts of two megadisasters in the most recent decade (Cyclone Nargis in 2008 and the 2010 Haitian earthquake) up from one megadisaster in 1996–2005 (the 2004 Indian Ocean Tsunami) [2]. The increasing disaster rate has disproportionately affected poorer nations and communities contributing to the downward spiraling effect on the economic, political, and public health conditions of several developing nations [1]. According to an analysis of the US Geological Survey data, since 1976 there have been 99 earthquakes of magnitude 7.0 or greater, 26 of them caused more than 1000 deaths, but only five of these disasters occurred in rich or middle-income countries [3]. Furthermore since 2001, while just 19% of violent earthquakes

P. Fugazzola (✉) · F. Coccolini · L. Ansaloni
Unit of General and Emergency Surgery, Bufalini Hospital, AUSL Romagna, Cesena, Italy

C. Merli
Unit of Emergency Medicine, Bufalini Hospital, AUSL Romagna, Cesena, Italy

E. Gamberini · V. Agnoletti
Unit of Anesthesia and Intensive Care, Bufalini Hospital, AUSL Romagna, Cesena, Italy

Y. Kluger et al. (eds.), *WSES Handbook of Mass Casualties Incidents Management*, Hot Topics in Acute Care Surgery and Trauma,
https://doi.org/10.1007/978-3-319-92345-1_15

worldwide have resulted in more than 1000 deaths, nearly 90% of them have been in poor countries [3, 4].

The Centre for Research on the Epidemiology of Disasters (CRED) created an Emergency Events Database (EM-DAT) that shows that also the severity of the impacts of natural hazards are directly related to income and development levels (Fig. 15.1). This is particularly evident for disaster mortality. The poorer the country, the higher the number of disaster deaths there are likely to be. Of the 1.35 million people killed by natural hazard over the past 20 years (more than half in earthquakes, with the remainder due to weather- and climate-related hazards), the overwhelming majority was in low- and middle-income countries, that have the highest numbers killed per disaster and per 100,000 population [2]. On average 327 people died per disaster in low-income countries in the past 20 years, almost five times more than the average toll in high-income countries (Fig. 15.2). Furthermore, none of the high-income countries which appear on the 2015 top ten list for economic losses from disaster appear among the countries suffering the highest disaster mortality [2]. Finally, the nonprofit GeoHazards International says that over the past few decades, rich countries have reduced mortality from earthquakes at a rate of ten times faster than poor countries [3].

Today some 613 million people live in 31 low-income countries. Many of these countries are either in post-conflict or conflict situations and lack the resources to account adequately for their disaster losses or to reduce their vulnerability to

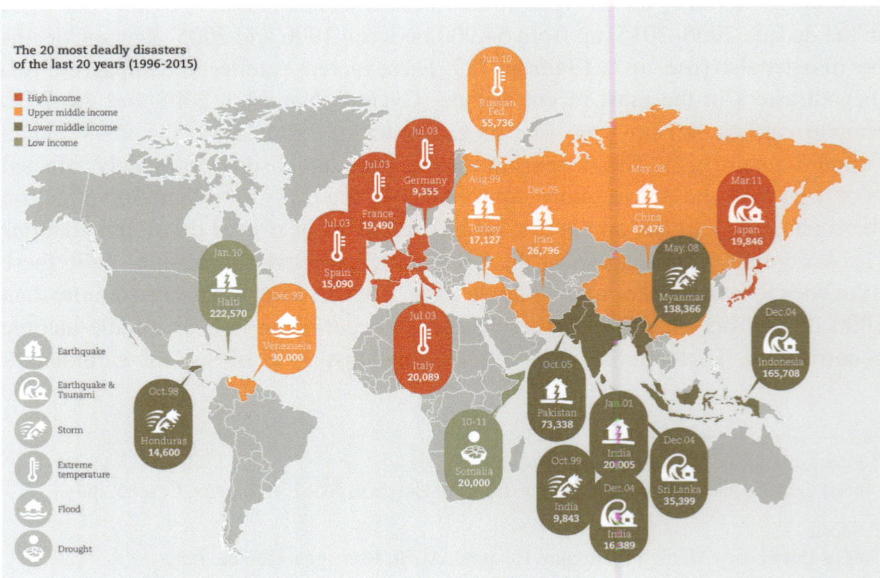
The 20 most deadly disasters
of the last 20 years (1996-2015)
High income
Upper middle income
Lower middle income
Low income
Earthquake
Earthquake & Tsunami
Storm
Extreme temperature
Flood
Drought
Jun.10 Russian Fed. 55,736
Jul.03 Germany 9,355
Jul.03 France 19,490
Jul.03 Spain 15,090
Jul.03 Italy 20,089
Aug.99 Turkey 17,127
Dec.03 Iran 26,796
May.08 China 87,476
Mar.11 Japan 19,846
May.08 Myanmar 138,366
Dec.04 Indonesia 165,708
Jan.10 Haiti 222,570
Dec.99 Venezuela 30,000
Oct.98 Honduras 14,600
10-11 Somalia 20,000
Oct.05 Pakistan 73,338
Jan.01 India 20,005
Oct.99 India 9,843
Dec.04 India 16,389
Dec.04 Sri Lanka 35,399

Fig. 15.1 The 20 most deadly disasters of the last 20 years (1996–2015). From *Poverty and death: disaster mortality 1996–2015* by the Centre for Reasearch on the Epidemiology of Disasters (CRED) [2]

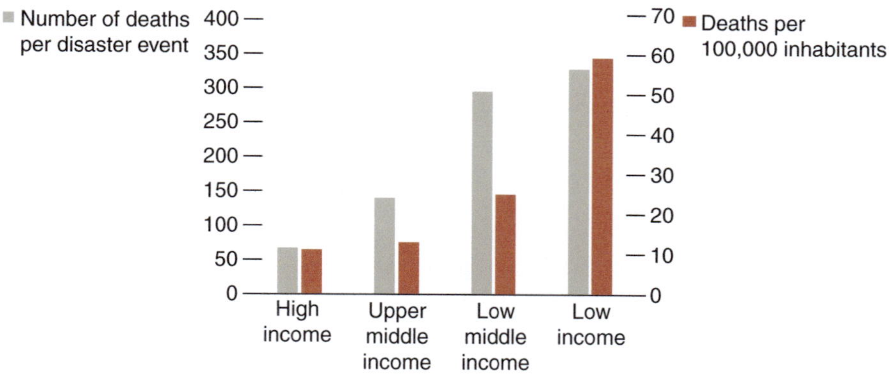

Fig. 15.2 Number of deaths per disaster event compared to the number of deaths per 100,000 inhabitans per income group, 1996–2015. From *Poverty and death: disaster mortality 1996–2015* by the Centre for Reasearch on the Epidemiology of Disasters (CRED) [2]

disasters. Thus disaster mortality in low-income countries is probably even higher than indicated in the EM-DAT [2].

15.2 Trauma Care in Low-Income Countries

Planning disaster preparedness and response for mass trauma is a huge undertaking for developing countries, because they often lack of an organized, efficient and effective trauma system. A trauma system is a regional coordination system that delivers the full range of care to all injured patients and it is integrated with the local public health system, making efficient use of health-care resources [1]. An efficient trauma system includes injury prevention, prehospital care, acute care facilities, and posthospital care. In low-income countries, there is gross disparity between trauma services in various portions of the country, there is no dedicated national lead agency to coordinate various components of trauma system, no mechanism for accreditation of trauma center exists, and there is an inappropriate resource allocation [1]. In fact, 90% of the world's trauma deaths occur in low- and middle-income countries (LMICs) [3].

In order to augment the capacity to provide trauma care in LMICs, in 2004, the World Health Organization (WHO) issued the Guidelines for Essential Trauma Care. The Guidelines outlines 11 essential trauma care services that should be available to every injured person around the world regardless of their country's income status (Table 15.1). These guidelines have been implemented in a number of countries and studies have shown some benefit in terms of trauma capacity [3]. However, to make improvements in trauma care in LMICs, health-care facilities had to be assessed in order to identify areas for targeted intervention. Then in 2007 the WHO's Global Initiative for Emergency and Essential Surgical Care developed the Tool for Situational Analysis to Assess Emergency and Essential Surgical Care (TSAAEESC)

Table 15.1 Essential trauma services

Obstructed airways are opened and maintained before hypoxia leads to death or permanent disability
Impaired breathing is supported until the injured person is able to breath adequately without assistance
Pneumothorax and hemothorax are promptly recognized and relieved
Bleeding (external or internal) is promptly stopped
Shock is recognized and treated with intravenous (IV) fluid replacement before irreversible consequences occur
The consequences of traumatic brain injury are lessened by timely decompression of space occupying lesions and by prevention of secondary brain injury
Intestinal and other abdominal injuries are promptly recognized and repaired
Potentially disabling extremity injuries are corrected
Potentially unstable spinal cord injuries are recognized and managed appropriately, including early immobilization
The consequences to the individual of injuries that result in physical impairment are minimized by appropriate rehabilitative services
Medications for the above services and for the minimization of pain are readily available when needed

to evaluate surgical capabilities of facilities in LMICs. The survey contains four section: infrastructures, human resources, interventions, emergency equipment and supplies. In response to the need for a more streamlined tool to evaluate surgical care, Surgeons Overseas modified TSAAEESC to create the simplified Personnel, Infrastructures, Procedures, Equipment and Supplies (PIPES). Afterwards, the need for a more specifically focused tool on emergency and critical care led to the development of the Emergency and Critical Care (EaCC) tool, which cover eight domains: infrastructures, human resources, training, drugs, equipment, routines, guidelines, support services [3]. These survey tools represent snapshots of workforce and hospital-based resources required to provide surgical care and, as trauma care relies on a subset of these resources, these assessments also provide information on components required for adequate trauma care [3].

Because substantial evidence exists in higher-income settings that the establishment of trauma system significantly decreases injury-related mortality, and some evidence suggests that this holds true in lower-resources setting, several studies tried to identify the more critical weaknesses in trauma systems of LMICs through the use of these tools [3]. Targeted corrective action addresses system weakness through initiatives that maximize benefit while minimizing costs [5]. In this setting, future efforts to improve trauma outcomes in these countries should address the following areas:

- *Prehospital care*. Prehospital trauma systems are rudimentary in many LMICs and currently an important proportion of prehospital care and transport is provided by layperson bystanders and commercial drivers. In fact, 80% of all trauma-related death in LMICs occurs in the prehospital setting [5]. It would be necessary to implement training programs for laypersons as first responders and to allocate material resources to them. Point-of-care interventions may have important survival benefits and hospital care may be futile without proper stabilization on the field [3]. The training for first responders should include external hemorrhage control, airway management, splinting, spinal immobilization, basic patient triage, and patient extrication [6]. The development of certified courses and of standardized treatment protocols is useful to improve standards of care. Because of the low level of literacy and health knowledge of layperson in LMICs, local physicians and health-care providers should teach courses in laypersons' native language to reduce language barriers [6]. One method to disseminating training materials and increasing basic first aid knowledge among laypersons is also by leveraging technology [6].

- *Primary care facilities availability in district hospital.* In LMICs, policy makers are rationally allocating their limited resources to higher-level referral centers. Surgical and trauma capacity is most limited in personnel, infrastructure, and procedures at rural and district facilities. In these settings, an ICU often consists of pressurized air or oxygen, but rarely mechanical ventilation or renal replacement therapy is present. Fifty percent of the patients have no monitors, necessary disposable material (EEG stickers, tubing), or electricity [7, 8]. Strengthening district hospitals, at list to a point of patient stabilization for transport to a referral center, is necessary [3]. Interventions should focus on increasing the number of surgical and anesthesia resources and personnel on rural areas [5].
- *Improvement in training of physicians and development of established protocol or checklist for the management of major trauma.* A trial in Trinidad and Tobago demonstrated a 50% decrease in injury mortality at a local tertiary care hospital after physicians attended the Advanced Trauma Life Support course. Similarly a project that trained paramedics in basic life support skills in Iraq and Cambodia dropped local trauma mortality rates from 22.6 to 13.7% in 2 years [2].
- *Posthospital care.* Rehabilitation services should also be addressed as trauma-associated morbidity remains significant and is likely to increase when mortality decreases [3].
- *Prevention programs.*

One potential pitfall in the improvement of trauma systems in LMICs is to attempt to replicate systems that have been successful in high-income countries. LMICs suffer from severe constraints of available resources, both in structural and human fields, and in these settings initiatives to improve trauma systems should be developed within the context of the resource limitations of the targeted region to decrease financial stress and inefficient resource allocation [9]. However, an estimated two million lives annually could be saved if injury mortality rates in LMICs were the same as that of high-income countries. The economic benefit from such a reduction in mortality and morbidity would be substantial, as road traffic injuries alone cost countries between 1 and 5% of their gross national product annually [3].

15.3 Mass Casualties in Low-Income Countries

The lack of a structured trauma system in low-income countries is reflected on the scarce ability to face a MCI or a disaster. During the Pakistan 2005 earthquake, approximately 75,000 people were killed and 70,000 were injured. In this occasion, lacking an integrated trauma system and a mass casualty preparedness, a "cluster approach" was adopted with several criticisms: failure to prioritize cross-cutting issues, weak information management, weak inter-cluster coordination, lack of centralized command, and inappropriate resource allocation (out of the 1698 patients air-ambulanced to Military Hospital Rawalpindi, only 50% actually required hospitalization, the rest either did not require inpatient care or were dead on arrival) [1]. Similarly during the earthquake that struck Haiti in 2010, the initial emergency response was delayed. The most important reason was that the earthquake destroyed the location of Haitian government offices and the main Haitian Hospital (University Hospital in Port-au-Prince). Many agencies around the world participated to improving resources, but this "clustered" medical teams had no way of knowing which hospitals had space or equipment, and communication between centers was absent for the first few days [1].

An analysis of the features of the early response to these and other disasters in low-income countries allowed to identify many criticisms [1, 8, 10]:

- Lack of national agency for disaster management
- Inadequate prehospital care, due to the lack of an efficient trauma system
- Lack of national high level trauma care facilities
- Lack of facility standard accreditations
- Lack of a pre-defined disaster management plan
- No disaster drills/simulations

Tight fiscal budget constraints, coupled with a lack of vision of the increasing probability of a disaster, have led governments to postpone progress on this issues to a later time. However, governments should consider that preparedness funding routinely returns five dollars for every dollar spent [3].

The Third UN World Conference on Disaster Risk Reduction, held in Sendai, Japan in 2015, resulted in the adoption of the Sendai Framework for Disaster Risk reduction 2015–2030. It identified four priorities for action for governments around the world [2]:

1. Understanding disaster risk in all its dimensions of vulnerability, capacity, exposure of persons and assets, hazard characteristics, and the environment
2. Strengthening disaster risk governance at the national, regional, and global levels to manage disaster risk
3. Investing in disaster risk reduction for resilience
4. Enhancing disaster preparedness for effective response and to "Build Back Better" in recovery, rehabilitation, and reconstruction

The actions necessary to implement MCIs management are often corollaries of the previously exposed actions necessary to develop an efficient trauma system. An effective trauma system may potentially manage mass casualty incident better [4]. However, an approach that works well in one country may work less well in another, and not all approaches are equally acceptable to all governments [9].

The Resource-Poor Setting panel of the Task Force for Mass Critical Care in 2014 outlined suggestions for capacity building and mitigation, preparedness, response, reconstruction, and recovery in MCIs in LMICs. Many of the capability building and mitigation suggestions are relevant to policy maker and health administration, whereas preparedness and response primarily relate to clinicians. The suggestions include capacity building in public health, education for families, community health-care workers and clinicians in addition to infrastructure support such as transportation and communication system. In order to mitigate the need for critical care, they suggest the development of simple triage tools, protocols, and care guidelines modified to resource limitations that can be used by health workers with limited clinical backgrounds. Furthermore, they stress the importance of the education and training of resuscitation, evacuation and transport of critically ill, expanding prehospital support in the community through education of medical and non-medical laypersons. They confirm the need of a minimal level of critical care at district or regional hospital facilities. Furthermore, local authorities should establish formal relationship with coalitions of academic medical centers, professional societies, governmental organization, and NGOs prior to an actual event in order to develop and maintain effective communication with the goal of assessing the need for assistance and of developing planning and preparation for potential disaster event [9, 11–15].

15.4 Take Home Message

- Low-income countries are the most exposed to disasters, because they have both the highest rate of disasters and the highest numbers killed per disaster and per 100,000 population.
- Low-income countries often lack an organized, efficient and effective trauma system and this is reflected on the scarce ability to face a MCI or a disaster.
- To make improvements in trauma care in LMICs, health-care facilities had to be assessed in order to identify areas for targeted intervention and initiatives that maximize benefit while minimizing costs.
- To make improvements in trauma care in LMICs, it would be necessary to implement training programs for laypersons as first responders, to allocate material resources to them, to improve in training of physicians, and to develop established protocol for the management of major trauma.
- Strengthening district hospitals, at list to a point of patient stabilization for transport to a referral center, is necessary.
- The actions necessary to implement MCIs management are often corollaries of the actions necessary to develop an efficient trauma system.

- The Resource-Poor Setting panel of the Task Force for Mass Critical Care in 2014 outlined suggestions for capacity building and mitigation, preparedness, response, reconstruction, and recovery in MCIs in LMICs. They involve both clinicians and policy maker.
- Governments of low-income country should invest in trauma-focused education and in disaster preparedness as the economic benefit from a reduction in mortality and morbidity would be substantial.

References

1. Khan FJ, Hassan M. Disaster planning for mass trauma care: implications for low income countries. Ital J Public Health. 2010;7(2):8.
2. United Nations Office for Disaster Risk Reduction (UNISDR), Centre for Research on the Epidemiology of Disasters (CRED). Poverty & death: disaster mortality 1996-2015. www.unisdr.org. [Online] https://www.unisdr.org/we/inform/publications/50589.
3. Holthaus E. Poor countries like Nepal are falling behind in preventing disaster. www.slate.it. [Online] http://www.slate.com/blogs/the_slatest/2015/04/26/nepal_earthquake_2015_poor_countries_like_haiti_are_underprepared_and_underfunded.html.
4. Aitken P, Leggat P. Considerations in mass casualty and disaster management. In: Blaivas M, editor. Emergency medicine. Rijeka: IntechOpen; 2012. ISBN: 978-953-51-0333-2. https://doi.org/10.5772/37361.
5. Wong EG, Gupta S, Deckelbaum DL, Razek T, Kushner AL. Prioritizing injury care: a review of trauma capacity in low and middle-income countries. J Surg Res. 2015;193(1):217–22. https://doi.org/10.1016/j.jss.2014.08.055. Epub 2014 Sep 4. Review.
6. Blair KJ, Paladino L, Shaw PL, Shapiro MB, Nwomeh BC, Swaroop M. Surgical and trauma care in low- and middle-income countries: a review of capacity assessments. J Surg Res. 2017;210:139–51. https://doi.org/10.1016/j.jss.2016.11.005. Epub 2016 Nov 10.
7. Geiling J, Burkle FM Jr, Amundson D, Dominguez-Cherit G, Gomersall CD, Lim ML, Luyckx V, Sarani B, Uyeki TM, West TE, Christian MD, Devereaux AV, Dichter JR, Kissoon N, Task Force for Mass Critical Care; Task Force for Mass Critical Care. Resource-poor settings: infrastructure and capacity building: care of the critically ill and injured during pandemics and disasters: CHEST consensus statement. Chest. 2014;146(4 Suppl):e156S–67S. https://doi.org/10.1378/chest.14-0744.
8. Razzak JA, Baqir SM, Khan UR, Heller D, Bhatti J, Hyder AA. Emergency and trauma care in Pakistan: a cross-sectional study of healthcare levels. Emerg Med J. 2015;32(3):207–13. https://doi.org/10.1136/emermed-2013-202590. Epub 2013 Oct 24.
9. Callese TE, Richards CT, Shaw P, Schuetz SJ, Paladino L, Issa N, Swaroop M. Trauma system development in low- and middle-income countries: a review. J Surg Res. 2015;193(1):300–7. https://doi.org/10.1016/j.jss.2014.09.040. Epub 2014 Oct 2. Review.
10. Blair KJ, Boeck MA, Gallardo Barrientos JL, Hidalgo López JL, Helenowski IB, Nwomeh BC, Shapiro MB, Swaroop M. Assessment of surgical and trauma capacity in Potosí, Bolivia. Ann Glob Health. 2017;83(2):262–73. https://doi.org/10.1016/j.aogh.2017.04.002. Epub 2017 May 24.
11. Callese TE, Richards CT, Shaw P, Schuetz SJ, Issa N, Paladino L, Swaroop M. Layperson trauma training in low- and middle-income countries: a review. J Surg Res. 2014;190(1):104–10. https://doi.org/10.1016/j.jss.2014.03.029. Epub 2014 Mar 20. Review.
12. Leow JJ, Brundage SI, Kushner AL, Kamara TB, Hanciles E, Muana A, Kamara MM, Daoh KS, Kingham TP. Mass casualty incident training in a resource-limited environment. Br J Surg. 2012;99(3):356–61. https://doi.org/10.1002/bjs.7762. Epub 2011 Dec 21.

13. Shah AA, Rehman A, Sayyed RH, Haider AH, Bawa A, Zafar SN, Zia-Ur-Rehman, Ali K, Zafar H. Impact of a predefined hospital mass casualty response plan in a limited resource setting with no pre-hospital care system. Injury. 2015;46(1):156–61. https://doi.org/10.1016/j.injury.2014.08.029. Epub 2014 Aug 19.
14. Latifi R, Gunn JK, Stroster JA, Zaimi E, Olldashi F, Dogjani A, Kerci M, Draçini X, Kuçani J, Shatri Z, Kociraj A, Boci A, Donaldson RI. The readiness of emergency and trauma care in low- and middle-income countries: a cross-sectional descriptive study of 42 public hospitals in Albania. Int J Emerg Med. 2016;9(1):26. Epub 2016 Oct 7.
15. Borgohain B, Khonglah T. Developing and organizing a trauma system and mass casualty management: some useful observations from the israeli trauma model. Ann Med Health Sci Res. 2013;3(1):85–9. https://doi.org/10.4103/2141-9248.109455.

16 Mass Casualties Incident: Education, Simulation, and Training

Itamar Ashkenazi, Kristina Lennquist Montán, and Sten Lennquist

16.1 Overview

Whenever a major incident occurs, an integrated and efficient response is necessary in order to make an impact on mortality and morbidity. This can only come about if the personnel involved are educated and trained in the unique procedures forethought to be necessary in the response to these events. The aim of this chapter is to discuss the challenges and different problems that may be encountered when educating and training medical personnel in this scenario. The focus is on events that may lead to a mass influx of patients suffering from injuries, whether following a terror attack (bombing, mass shooting, truck stampeding into a crowd), mass gathering disaster, mass transport accident, or an industrial disaster without an overt toxicologic component.

The main challenge facing the health system is how to achieve preparedness for an event for which the circumstances and scope are not fully known. Risk assessment is carried out in order to determine possible consequences of realistic threats [1]. Contingency plans should be developed for possible scenarios. These should identify potential responders, potential procedures, and potential tools necessary to carry out the plan. No matter which component of the response is being planned for,

I. Ashkenazi (✉)
Hillel Yaffe Medical Center, Hadera, Israel

K. L. Montán
Department of Public Health Sciences, Traumacenter Karolinska, Karolinska University Hospital, Karolinska Institute, Solna, Sweden
e-mail: kristina.lennquist-montan@ki.se

S. Lennquist
International MRMID-Association, University of Linköping, Linköping, Sweden
e-mail: Lennquist@telia.com

Y. Kluger et al. (eds.), *WSES Handbook of Mass Casualties Incidents Management*, Hot Topics in Acute Care Surgery and Trauma,
https://doi.org/10.1007/978-3-319-92345-1_16

there is no alternative to prior education and training of those responders who will be responsible for carrying out the task once the calamity strikes [2].

Major incidents lead not only to injuries and to deaths, but also to disruptions in infrastructure and logistics all of which may affect the response. The response to these events will involve not only the health system, but also other sectors, such as security forces, other rescue services, and different government agencies. Different organizations need to learn how to work together in order not to interfere with one another during a real event. This can only be done if the aims of the different sectors involved are made known and prioritized before the event occurs. Members of the health system, for example, need to learn how to cooperate with the police and firefighters [3]. Simulations should be instituted in order to assess whether different organizations have indeed implemented the necessary tools to allow a coordinated response [4–6].

The medical response to major incidents in itself is also complex. Members of the health system that need to be educated and trained include medical first responders, hospital first receivers such as physicians and nurses, and health care institution support personnel such as janitors, hospital administrators, laboratory personnel, radiology technicians, and security personnel [7]. Members of each of these sectors have different responsibilities within the medical chain of response during a crisis. The educational content and intensity of training for each sector will be different. Identifying response components that can be incorporated into daily professional practices together with just-in-time training is one strategy to create a sustainable mechanism allowing members of the health care delivery system the ability to respond properly during the crisis [7]. Furthermore, identifying those critical components that are not part of the daily professional practices foretells which components will probably fail during the event [8]. These should be the elements most emphasized during simulation sessions.

While the need to educate and train for a possible event is clear, there are still many deficiencies to overcome. It is not uncommon to encounter hospitals without detailed disaster plans and without active disaster committees [9, 10]. Challenges to education and training include lack of time and lack of staff devoted to training. Training is not prioritized due to absence of ubiquitous support, incentives, or requirements among health professions [11]. Most of the education and training done is fragmentized by the different professions involved and even within each profession, the teaching and training of the different proficiencies are fragmentized. Infrequent exercises lead to personnel's uncertainty concerning their role during a real event [8, 12]. These problems are further complicated by myriad of solutions that exist for similar problems creating a chaos between similar training systems, for example, triage [13–15]. Seldom are all the components of the chain of response trained together [2]. Current available options for training are limited by lack of realism, prohibitive expense, and lack of assessment tools [16].

16.2 Types of Education, Simulation, and Training

Extensive literature exists on different techniques employed in educating and training possible responders in their role of action during a mass casualty incident (Table 16.1). These may be technologically simple such as paper-based exercises

Table 16.1 Training tools and possibilities

Possibilities	Advantages	Disadvantages
Classroom based		
Paper-based exercises	Not expensive	No evaluation of the system
Didactic Lectures	Large number of trainees	
Computer based		
Computer simulations	Dynamic	Expensive
Virtual reality	Quantitative measurements	
	Reproducible	
Injured patient simulators		
Sims	Dynamic	Expensive
Live actors (inexperienced)	Have been incorporated in	Inexperienced actors may
Live actors (experienced)	large-scale exercises	confuse the trainees
Exercises		
Table-top	Interactive	May not test specific
	Inexpensive	logistical issues
	Reproducible	
Small-scale injury tag based	Inexpensive	Limited number of trainees
	May be used as surprise drill	Dynamics is limited
Large-scale injury tag based	Large number of trainees	Expensive
		Dynamics is limited

Adapted from Ashkenazi et al. [17]

and didactic lessons or technologically complex such as interactive virtual simulations and high fidelity human patient simulators [18–22]. Didactic lessons, large-scale exercises, and pilot demonstration projects enable education and training of a large number of people at the same time [23]. Other techniques such as virtual simulators may be more limited in the number of people who can participate in any one session.

The different techniques are usually targeted at specific sectors of responders such as medical first responders and other health care personnel. Some efforts are less selective and involve medical students who may find themselves in the future, during their professional life, responding to a mass casualty incident [23, 24]. Training courses have been developed to teach non-medical personnel-specific skill, such as triage skills course for non-medical members of other rescue services [25, 26]. Courses have been developed even for the lay public in order to make these ready to assist if in case a mass casualty event occurs [27]. Some of the skills needed in order to respond may need refreshment. For this purpose, some of the courses include a short-term “last minute” training session [28]. Alternatively, aide memoirs may be used as last minute reminders [22].

Many of these educational courses and training sessions include an element of evaluation. Many base their evaluation on Likert charts, where student participants evaluate their perceived competencies before and after the course [3, 29–31]. Other tools used for evaluation include surveys, pretests, and post-tests [8, 32]. Responders' knowledge and confidence can be reevaluated several months later [26, 31]. Some forms of training allow quantifiable data to be collected, such as triage accuracy [25, 26, 33]. Virtual reality scenarios allow recording errors, delays and completion of action, as well as assessment of non-technical skills [16].

More important is the content of most of these educational efforts. Depending on the specific training course, these include, among others, basic disaster life support techniques, prehospital trauma life support, advanced trauma life support, different triage techniques, and different procedures that might be needed, such as proper tourniquet placement [30, 34]. It is clear that the myriad courses that exist, each based on the education of specific skills and aimed at specific sectors, raise doubt about the real value of these courses in training the system to be prepared for a mass casualty incident. Many of these present themselves as educational initiatives meant to improve response to mass casualty incidents. Whether this is true is questionable.

Once the risks are realized and the contingency plans thought out, it is necessary to evaluate who should be educated and trained to respond for these events. Splitting the plan into different areas of responsibility and allocating key personnel from each area to propose the most appropriate strategies to fulfill the tasks under their responsibility is key in producing a plan that is feasible. This approach also serves the purpose of education since collaborating with key personnel to produce parts of the plan will enhance their own performance when the need arises Collaborating with key personnel will also help identify other human resources and procedures needed to carry out the role within each of the areas of responsibility. Any of the methods mentioned above is legitimate in training potential responders. Familiarity with the area of responsibility will help key personnel define which responders need more training and which tasks or skills are not employed routinely and therefore need strengthening.

While the model proposed above has many benefits, it should be emphasized that fragmentation of preparedness needs to be complemented by a process that examines how the different components of the system work together. Educational and training sessions of specific skills may be common. However, training of larger parts of the system is infrequent, becoming less common as the number of potential sector participants increases. In Israel, for example, the prehospital emergency system trains alone and different hospitals each train individually for mass casualty incidents. Over the last two decades, only few exercises were dedicated to test both the hospital and prehospital systems together. Joint training of the medical system with other rescue agencies and security forces is rare and usually limited to table-top exercises involving managerial positions.

A different approach is taken by the developers of the Medical Response to Major Incidents (MRMI) postgraduate course (Fig. 16.1) [5, 35]. The main idea behind the course is to introduce students to the whole chain of medical response: prehospital system, hospital system, and regional medical command. The students learn the theory and practice of the main sites and functions within the system. Two large table-top exercises constitute the backbone of the course where the students need to treat multiple victims following a major event. The injured victims are based on a real scenario. The real consumption of time and resources for every decision made is clearly illustrated, and also the consequences of the decisions with regard to mortality and complications, giving the trainees proper feedback with regard to the accuracy of the decisions on all levels in the chain of response.

Though the emphasis of the course is medical response, members of other rescue agencies and security forces participate. The students who work in the different stations learn to communicate their needs with other stations, whether these are

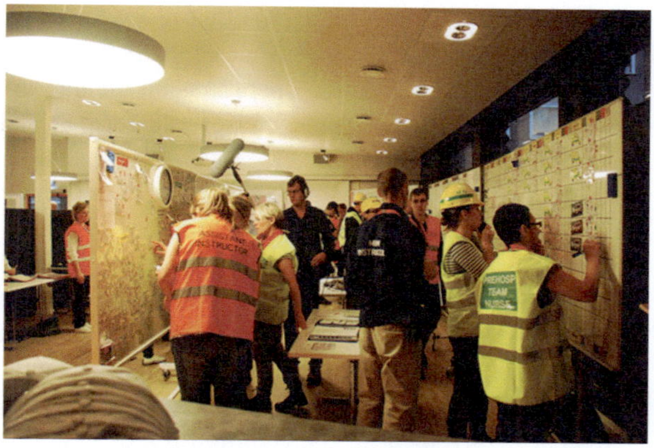

Fig. 16.1 Students training in primary and secondary triage in a mass casualty incident table-top exercise held in Karolinska Institute, Stockholm 2013 (courtesy of International MRMID-Association)

medical or pertaining to the other non-medical agencies responding to the event. Since the injured victims represent patients with specific injuries and specific needs, the medical system response can be measured. Impact of different approaches adopted by one component of the system may raise problems that will be experienced downstream within the chain. For example, minimal or no treatment on a scene with prolonged transport times will lead to increased mortality of patients with airway problems during transport. On the other extreme, an over-cautious policy of intubation on the scene will negatively affect the workup possibilities of multiple patients once these are admitted to the hospital. The course lectures are supplemented by manuals and the Medical Response to Major Incidents and Disasters textbook that serves as a guidebook for this course [36]. The accuracy of the course for its purpose has been scientifically validated on a large number of trainees from many different countries [32].

Large-scale exercises enable training large numbers of staff in their role usually within their natural environment. Apart from testing decision-making, large-scale exercises have an added benefit of testing certain logistical issues that cannot be otherwise reproduced within other training formats. For example, large-scale exercises help identify obstacles in patient flow both in the scene and in the hospitals. In the setup of the hospital, problems with simultaneous inflow of a number of ambulances with patients can be appreciated as well as mobilization of patients between the different sites within the hospital itself. The efficacy of the method for rapid patient registration can also be assessed. This is crucial since different aspects of vital treatment of severely injured patients rely on proper patient identification.

Though allowing to train simultaneously the staff within their natural environment, large-scale exercises do not offer a comprehensive solution for MCI education and training. Patient flow may be assessed in the hospitals' emergency departments or radiology departments, but cannot be reproduced in the intensive care units and within the operating rooms. Furthermore, the role of large-scale exercises should be re-examined in a reality where the medical system, though expected to be prepared to respond to a calamity, is mainly judged by its ability to maintain economic viability. In order to be effective, most, if not all those involved in the response, should be relieved from other tasks during the large-scale exercise itself. Large-scale exercises demand from hospitals to limit economic activities such as outpatient clinics and routine operations on the day of the exercise. The economic losses entailed by large-scale exercises transform these into an unattractive solution for hospital administrations.

Table-top exercises may reproduce most of the components trained in large-scale exercises. Those activities in major incident response that have to be tested and trained "live" to secure function can be done in small-scale exercises involving selected individual units. Planning and integration of both table-top exercises and small-scale exercises are essential in order to produce an effective system for education and training that can be repeated as necessary with minimal constraints on the medical system.

Recent involvement of the coalition forces in conflicts in Iraq and Afghanistan has created a new dimension for education and training [37]. The experience in treatment of war-like injuries within the civilian sector is limited. Nevertheless, use of bombs and high-velocity automatic guns are commonly used by perpetrators aiming at causing incidents with as many casualties as possible. New courses are being created with the aim to introduce civilian physicians with this type of injuries. The realization that the types of injuries that may be encountered following terror attacks will be different from those commonly encountered in everyday trauma scenarios should be emphasized if we wish to make an impact on survival.

16.3 A Rationale Approach to MCI Education and Training

It is time to reevaluate the current approach to MCI education and training that has created a chaotic environment of multiple endeavors that vary in their aims and contents across geographical regions and rescue systems within the same region. Realization that the medical response to major incidents demands a synchronized approach across the medical system as well as effective collaboration with other rescue services, security forces, and government agencies should be emphasized. Current efforts should be maintained, but prioritized according to their contribution to preparedness according to the regional plan. We therefore suggest:

1. Link the educational effort with the regional plan.

   As explained above, involving responders in the planning phase contributes not only to the feasibility of the plan, but also to the education of those who will lead the response to the event.
2. Education and training should target the whole chain of response. This should be supplemented by education of specific skills needed by specific responders.

   While effective planning demands fragmentation of the plan into its components, effective execution demands the plan to be evaluated as a whole. Training the whole chain of response will identify the gaps in the plan, many of which tend to occur in between components executed by different sectors of the response.

3. Identify the components of the plan that rely on procedures done on routine basis and those which are not.

   The plan is as good as its weakest link. Procedures that are not in common use will fail if responders are not acquainted with these. Involving the responders in the planning phase is one strategy to increase acquaintance of responders with their role. Identifying those uncommon procedures helps identify which procedures need frequent training.
4. Define for each education and training undertaking a set of learning objectives that corresponds to objective of the plan.

Evaluation of regional readiness demands periodic review of the plan against the learning objectives of available educational and training efforts. Gaps identified should be fixed with most appropriate method of education and training.

Conflicts of Interest Sten Lennquist and Kristina Lennquist Montán are the developers of the MACSIM® (www.macsim.se) simulation system in use by different organizations across Europe, in Thailand and in the Ukraine for training in the management of mass casualty incidents. The MACSIM simulation system is the basis of the Medical Response to Major Incidents (MRMI) postgraduate course, which also was developed by Sten Lennquist and Kristina Lennquist Montán and now is owned by the International MRMID-Association, which is a non-profit organization (www.mrmi.eu). Sten Lennquist was also the developer of the Emergo Train System, the processor of MACSIM. Itamar Ashkenazi is the developer of the smart injury tag system in use by the Israeli Homefront Command in large-scale exercises that test Israeli hospitals' preparedness.

References

1. Aven T, Guikema S. On the concept and definition of terrorism risk. Risk Anal. 2015;35(12):2162–71.
2. Lennquist S, Lennquist MK. Education and training. In: Lennquist S, editor. Medical response to major incidents and disasters. Berlin: Spinger; 2012. p. 379–98.
3. Jones J, Kue R, Mitchell P, Eblan G, Dyer KS. Emergency medical services response to active shooter incidents: provider comfort level and attitudes before and after participation in a focused response training program. Prehosp Disaster Med. 2014;29(4):350–7.
4. Balch D, Taylor C, Rosenthal D, Bausch C, Warner D, Morris R. Shadow Bowl 2003: a collaborative exercise in community readiness, agency cooperation, and medical response. Telemed J E Health. 2004;10(3):330–42.
5. Lennquist Montán K, Hreckovski B, Dobson B, Ortenwall P, Montán C, Khorram-Manesh A, Lennquist S. Development and evaluation of a new simulation model for interactive training of the medical response to major incidents and disasters. Eur J Trauma Emerg Surg. 2014;40(4):429–43.
6. Khorram-Manesh A, Lönroth H, Rotter P, Wilhelmsson M, Aremyr J, Berner A, Nero Andersson A. Carlström E. Non-medical aspects of civilian-military collaboration in management of major incidents. Eur J Trauma Emerg Surg. https://doi.org/10.1007/s00068-017-0778-6.
7. Blumenthal DJ, Bader JL, Christensen D, Koerner J, Cuellar J, Hinds S, Crapo J, Glassman E, Potter AB, Singletary L. A sustainable training strategy for improving health care following a catastrophic radiological or nuclear incident. Prehosp Disaster Med. 2014;29(1):80–6.
8. Radestad M, Lennquist Montán K, Ruter A, Castren M, Svensson L, Gryth D, Fossum B. Attitudes towards and experience of the use of triage tags in major incidents: a mixed method study. Prehosp Disaster Med. 2016;31(4):376–85.

9. Djalali A, Della Corte F, Foletti M, Ragazzoni L, Ripoll Gallardo A, Lupescu O, Arcuelo C, von Arnin G, Friedel T, Ashkenazi M, Fischer P, Hreckovski B, Khorram-Manesh A, Komadina R, Lechner K, Patru C, Burkle FM Jr, Ingrassia PL. Art of disaster preparedness in European union: a survey on the health systems. PLoS Curr. 2014;6. pii: ecurrents.dis.56cf1c5c1b0deae1595a48e294685d2f. https://doi.org/10.1371/currents.dis.56cf1c5c1b0deae1595a48e294685d2f.
10. Bin Shalhoub AA, Khan AA, Alaska YA. Evaluation of disaster preparedness for mass casualty incidents in private hospital in central Saudi Arabia. Saudi Med J. 2017;38(3):302–6.
11. Walsh L, Craddock H, Gulley K, Strauss-Riggs K, Schor KW. Building health care system capacity: training health care professionals in disaster preparedness health care coalitions. Prehosp Disaster Med. 2015;30(2):123–30.
12. Risavi BL, Terrell MA, Lee W, Holsten DL Jr. Prehospital mass-casualty triage training – written versus moulage scenarios: how much do EMS providers retain. Prehosp Disaster Med. 2013;28(3):251–6.
13. Lennquist MK. Triage. In: Lenquist S, editor. Medical response to major incidents and disasters. Berlin: Spinger; 2012. p. 63–75.
14. Lennquist Montán K, Khorram-Manesh A, Ortenwall P, Lennquist S. Comparative study of physiological and anatomical triage in major incidents using a new simulation model. Am J Disaster Med. 2011;6(5):289–98.
15. Arcos Gonzales P, Castro Delgado R, Cuartas Alvarez T, Gorijo Gonzalo G, Martinez Monzon C, Pelaez Corres N, Rodriguez Soler A, Turegano Fuentes F. The development and features of the Spanish prehospital advanced triage method (META) for mass casualty incidents. Scand J Trauma Resusc Emerg Med. 2016. Apr;29(24):63. https://doi.org/10.1186/s13049-016-0255-y.
16. Pucher PH, Batrick N, Taylor D, Chaudery M, Cohen D, Darzi A. Virtual-world hospital simulation for real-world disaster response: design and validation of a virtual reality simulator for mass casualty incident management. J Trauma Acute Care Surg. 2014;77(2):315–21.
17. Ashkenazi I, Ohana A, Azaria A, Gelfer A, Nave C, Deutch Z, Gens I, Fadlon M, Dahan Y, Rapaport L, Kishkinov D, Bar A, Tal-Or E, Vakinin N, Blumenfeld A, Kessl B, Alfici R, Olsha O, Michaelson M. Assessement of hospital disaster plans for conventional mass casualty incidents following terrorist explosions using a live exercise based upon the real data of actual patients. Eur J Trauma Emerg Surg. 2012;38(2):113–7.
18. Colander B, Green B, Millo Y, Shamloo C, Donnellan J, DeAtley C. Development of an "all hazard" hospital disaster preparedness training course utilizing multi-modality teaching. Prehosp Disaster Med. 2008;23(1):63–7.
19. Vincent DS, Sherstyuk A, Burgess L, Connolly KK. Teaching mass casualty triage skills using immersive three-dimensional virtual reality. Acad Emerg Med. 2008;15(11):1160–5.
20. Vincent DS, Burgess L, Berg BW, Connolly KK. Teaching mass casualty triage skills using iterative multimanikin simulations. Prehosp Emerg Care. 2009;13(2):241–6.
21. Leow JJ, Brudage SI, Kushner AL, Kamara TB, Hanciles E, Muana A, Kamara MM, Daoh KS, Kingham TP. Mass casualty incident training in a resource-limited environment. Br J Surg. 2012;99(3):356–61.
22. Cuttance G, Dansie K, Tayner T. Paramedic application of a triage sieve: a paper-based exercise. Prehosp Disaster Med. 2017;32(1):3–13.
23. Jorm C, Roberts C, Lim R, Roper J, Skinner C, Robertson J, Gentilcore S, Osomanski A. A large-scale mass casualty simulation to develop the non-technical skills medical students require for collaborative teamwork. BMC Med Educ. 2016;16:83. https://doi.org/10.1186/s12909-016-0588-2.
24. Rivkind AI, Faroja M, Mintz Y, Pikarsky AJ, Zamir G, Elazary R, Abu-Gazala M. Combating terror: a new paradigm in student trauma education. J Trauma Acute Care Surg. 2015;78(2):415–21.
25. Lee CW, McLeod SL, Peddle MB. First responder accuracy using SALT after brief initial training. Prehosp Disaster Med. 2015;30(5):447–51.
26. Nilsson A, Aslund K, Lampi M, Nilsson H, Jonson CO. Improved and sustained triage skills in firemen after a short training intervention. Scand J Trauma Resusc Emerg Med. 2015;23:81. https://doi.org/10.1186/s13049-015-0162-7.

27. Goolsby C, Branting A, Chen E, Mack E, Olsen C. Just-in-Time to save lives: a pilot study of layperson tourniquet application. Acad Emerg Med. 2015;22(9):1113–7. https://doi.org/10.1111/acem.12742. Epub 2015 Aug 20.
28. Badiali S, Giugni A, Marcis L. Testing the START triage protocol: can it improve the ability of non-medical personnel to better triage patients during disasters and mass casualties incidents? Disaster Med Public Health Prep. 2017;11(3):305–9.
29. Heinrichs WL, Youngblood P, Harter P, Kusumoto L, Dev P. Training healthcare personnel for mass-casualty incidents in a virtual emergency. Prehosp Disaster Med. 2010;25(5):424–32.
30. Kuhls DA, Chestovich PJ, Coule P, Carrison DM, Chua CM, Wora-Urai N, Kanchanrin T. Basic Disaster Life Support (BDLS) training improves first responder confidence to face mass-casualty incidents in Thailand. Prehosp Disaster Med. 2017;13:1–9. https://doi.org/10.1017/S1049023X17006550.
31. Bank I, Khalil E. Are pediatric physicians more knowledgeable and confider to respond to a pediatric disaster after an experimental learning experience? Prehosp Disaster Med. 2016;31(5):551–6.
32. Lennquist Montán K, Örtenwall P, Lennquist S. Assessment of the accuracy of the MRMI-course for interactive training of the medical response to major incidents and disasters. Am J Disaster Med. 2015;10(2):93–107.
33. Cicero MX, Whitfill T, Overly F, Baird J, Walsh B, Yarzebski J, Riera A, Adelgais K, Meckler GD, Baum C, Cone DC, Auerback M. Pediatric disaster triage: multiple simulation curriculum improves prehospital care providers' assessment skills. Prehosp Emerg Care. 2017;21(2):201–8.
34. Lampi M, Junker J, Berggren P, Jonson CO, Vikstrom T. Pre-hospital triage performance after standardized trauma courses. Scand J Trauma Resusc Emerg Med. 2017;25(1):53.
35. MRMI. http://mrmi.eu/. Accessed 1 Oct 2017.
36. Lennquist S, editor. Medical response to major incidents and disasters-a practical guide for all medical staff. Berlin: Springer; 2012.
37. Remick KN, Shackelford S, Oh JS, Seery JM, Grabo D, Chovanes J, Gross KR, Nessen SC, Tai NR, Rickard RF, Elster E, Schwab CW. Surgeon preparedness for mass casualty events: adapting essential military surgical lessons for the home front. Am J Disaster Med. 2016;11(2):77–87.

Debriefing Session: The Process of Self-Evaluation

17

Seema Yalamanchili, Sophie E. J. Hardy, and Christopher Aylwin

17.1 Purpose

Over the past decade, the global growth in both terror attacks and road traffic accidents has contributed to the apparent increase in incidence of major incidents worldwide [1, 2]. In major incidents, the location, number, severity or type of live casualties require the extraordinary mobilisation of resources [3, 4]. This can test emergency systems which may not be well practised in dealing with these events. Learning from the organisational performance accompanying a major incident gives the organisation an increased ability to anticipate, prepare, and respond to similar tests of function in future, thus increasing its resilience [38]. Alongside preventive measures, such as optimisation of health services, learning from debrief can reduce the morbidity and mortality incurred in such events. Effective debrief allows a review of emergency system performance and, in carefully selected cases, a forum for the initial address of the psychological trauma staff may have experienced.

17.2 Organisational Systems Learning

The debrief underpins the learning process at organisational, team and individual levels. Current debriefing educational theory has its basis in Kolb's learning cycle, wherein adult learners use experiences to modify their performance and goals [5].

The collective knowledge that contributes to a major incident plan amongst emergency services combines the specialist knowledge of certain divisions within the

S. Yalamanchili · C. Aylwin (✉)
St Mary's Hospital, London, UK
e-mail: christopher.aylwin@nhs.net

S. E. J. Hardy
St George's Hospital, London, UK

Y. Kluger et al. (eds.), *WSES Handbook of Mass Casualties Incidents Management*, Hot Topics in Acute Care Surgery and Trauma,
https://doi.org/10.1007/978-3-319-92345-1_17

organisation with knowledge developed by the organisation through shared experience [6]. Organisational learning revolves around implementing optimal learning from both positive and negative experiences through controlled and uncontrolled mechanisms, i.e. formal and informal debrief [7]. Through this learning cycle, an organisation is able to behave dynamically and innovate to overcome previous barriers to optimal performance and to anticipate additional difficulties to plan ahead.

Following a major incident, emergency services have a responsibility to return to full operational capacity, but also to take stock and analyse important lessons to identify both positive practice and areas for improvement. Without this pivotal step, the organisation runs the risk of repeating similar errors from previous events.

Some literature around organisational learning suggests that it takes time and if any significant gains are to be recognised, it should be viewed as an effective strategy over the longer term [8]. Conversely other authors have argued that this learning curve can be bypassed, at least in part, through effective data sharing [9]. If data from major incidents are shared globally, then a much wider repertoire of learning outcomes can be drawn upon for institutions around the world to make more responsive plans without necessarily having had to deal with vast numbers of major incidents themselves. Industry studies suggest that public sector organisations can tend towards working in silos and be slower to embrace dynamic change than their private sector counterparts. Given that emergency services are frequently public sector entities, it is important that frontline workers and strategic leaders in emergency services remain mindful of the need to evolve [9].

17.3 Human Performance Optimisation in Health Systems

Despite the growth in organisational learning in emergency systems in recent years, similar advances in team-based learning have been less forthcoming [10]. However, with the presence of multiple casualties it is important that the teams at the forefront of rescue, retrieval and delivery of clinical care are versed in learning processes.

Much of the published work around human performance in emergency clinical teams has arisen from reporting and debrief following critical incidents and simulation. Major incidents can be viewed as a form of critical incident [11]. Although not on the same scale as major incidents, critical incidents also pertain relatively rare occurrences of an emergency nature which test the skills of the teams involved. Accordingly, there is a rich body of knowledge from this field that can be extrapolated, modified and applied to the systems and culture around major incidents. Furthermore, good debriefing technique requires time to be developed as a skill so where possible, experienced facilitators in debrief in critical incidents and simulation should be used to assist with leading major incident debriefs [12].

17.3.1 Human Factors

The human factors approach has its roots in safety critical industries, such as aviation, and has been adopted within military and civilian emergency services to fortify performance [10]. It acknowledges human limitations and that through understanding of human behaviour and interactions with the surrounding systems, human frailties can be minimised to reduce negative sequelae [13]. The clinical human factors approach aims to enhance performance through an understanding of the effects of teamwork, tasks, equipment, workspace, culture and organisations on human behaviour and abilities and the application of that knowledge in the clinical setting [14].

In the context of a major incident, systems are stressed and although major incident plans may be in place, their execution is dependent on the performance of staff. It is therefore essential that any planning and debrief incorporate these considerations to optimise human performance. Reflective teams are more likely to improve performance and if conducted appropriately, debrief can improve both individual and team performance by up to 25% [10, 15]. Therefore during the debrief, teams must not only reflect how performance matched up to planned objectives, but also how non-technical skills could be built upon to improve the situational awareness, cognition, interpersonal communication and leadership of team members.

17.3.2 Psychosocial Considerations

The ensuing emotions following a major incident can be detrimental to frontline staff who have been exposed to difficult and potentially overwhelming circumstances not uncommonly involving serious injury or death. Following any disaster or major incident, the psychosocial aim is prevention of negative mental health outcomes so debriefs must take a humane, empathetic but competent approach with attention given to the thoughts and feelings of those involved.

Frustration or a sense of injustice may fuel anger either directed at oneself or at others. Guilt may occur when individuals feel more could have been done. For some individuals, a sense of helplessness or worry about a repeat event might lead to ongoing fear and diminished mood [16]. In extreme cases, staff can develop post-traumatic stress disorder (PTSD), an adjustment disorder characterised by a prolonged reaction to the trauma including re-experiencing of the event through nightmares and flashbacks [17]. PTSD is rare, but more common medium to long-term mental health problems include anxiety, depression, breakdown in interpersonal relationships and substance abuse [18]. Following major incidents there is evidence that the way psychosocial reactions are managed can define the extent and effect of community recovery and therefore action should be taken to not cause secondary psychosocial harm [19].

Educational debriefing focuses on learning from experience and differs from psychosocial debriefing. As debrief became popular in the 1980s, elements of educational and psychological debriefing became mixed together [20]. There remains an ongoing debate as to the psychosocial benefits of debrief over potential harm. This stems from a paucity of data and difficulty making broad interpretations of historical studies which vary in debrief aim, format, participant type, indication and context [21].

If handled poorly, the sharing of personal experience in an open forum can have detrimental effects and further traumatise individuals, especially if conducted at the wrong time and by untrained personnel [22]. Debrief around major incidents cannot be divorced from the necessary critique, but the use of positive confrontation and good judgement can counter the potential development of an intimidating atmosphere. Additionally, work around debriefing staff groups that have been briefed together prior to dealing with an incident has shown positive psychological effects [23].

The International Society for Traumatic Stress Studies' current guidelines on debrief acknowledge that whilst there is limited evidence for preventing mental health problems, debrief has a role in improving organisational learning and morale as well as helping to screen for those with mental health difficulties. They also stipulate that debriefs must have a clear structure and be conducted by trained facilitators [24]. Rather than psychosocial debrief, mental health professionals now place emphasis on psychological first aid which centres around informal approach of compassion and support from friends, family and colleagues to provide social, physical and welfare needs without necessarily discussing the emotional trauma from the incident in the acute setting [24].

17.4 Debrief in Training and Education

Although the frequency of major incidents is increasing, it remains a relatively rare occurrence. In order to increase learning opportunities around major incidents, various emergency services provide training courses and simulation. These take place on both single agency and multi-agency levels. Given its key role in learning, debrief features strongly in both these educational tools. Courses, such as Major Incident Medical Management and Support (MIMMS), discuss its importance and format. MIMMS even includes a workshop dedicated to major incident debriefing [4]. Training exercises vary in scale which can be costly but offer an excellent means of developing organisational capacity. They often have a significant debriefing component and learning points derived from simulation exercises can be used to improve major incident plans without having to expose the organisation to an actual major incident.

17.5 Briefing, Debrief and Documentation

During a major incident, there is a continual process of briefing to determine task allocation and execution, followed by debriefing before services begin to recover [25]. Thus, the work from the debrief represents the final part of an audit cycle that must be recorded to ensure that subsequently reports can be generated for sharing, major incident plans modified and information provided in the case of any judicial inquiry.

As the outputs from debrief can particularly augment organisational learning, incident commanders should consider the plans for debrief early. These plans are ideally disseminated promptly and in a protracted incident the debriefing process may even begin at an early stage, in order that any staff involved only at the initial phase may inform those working on the later response. Early instruction of these plans also avoids the operational pressures of returning normal service eclipsing the need for an effective debriefing process.

Documentation of debriefing activities should occur for legal purposes and for potential public inquiry into operational performance as well as organisational learning. A debrief should generate the following documents:

Minutes of debrief

- **Incident logs**: A record of events as they occurred in real time. This may be documented manually or by other means such as audio and later transcribed.
- **Organisation report**: It demonstrates where the institution's response was effective and where it was not. On an objective level, it should establish why this was the case and recommend ways to improve the future response. It should resist criticising individual actions.

Lessons identified

- **Action plan**: It gives a list of actions that have arisen as a result of the debrief. This should include revision of the major incident plan based on lessons identified. A named individual should be responsible for completing each action within an agreed time frame [26].

Processes should also be put in place for both storage and sharing of records both within the organisation and with other agencies. Records need to adhere to data protection laws including anonymisation and safe storage.

17.6 Debrief in Other Emergency Services

Debriefing is a fundamental organisational process and its use around major incidents is particularly embedded in those agencies who provide the immediate emergency response, namely police and fire services and prehospital medical organisations. The general principles discussed above are universal and have been adopted across these agencies with appropriate modifications for their specialist purposes, but ultimately all aim to identify lessons, which can be learnt to improve practice in the future.

As outlined, the military have distinguished history and culture of debriefing [10]. In the United Kingdom, the College of Policing describes standards for debrief but also provides a dedicated team who apply a professional structure to debriefing. Any police force within the country has access to their expertise to support them should a major incident occur [11]. Due to the frequency with which they attend major incidents, as not all major incidents generate casualties, they also have a body of staff trained in formal debriefing technique. Given the expertise of these services, health organisations could look to these groups to learn good debrief practice.

17.6.1 Multi-agency Debrief

Debriefing occurs at different levels and in major incidents there is a requirement for multi-agency debriefs. At this level it involves planners, facilitators and agency leads. The success of the incident response is a function of the combined efforts of the different agencies, including emergency transport, security and health services, and the degree to which they can communicate and cooperate. Multi-agency debriefing may take place through meetings organised by agency leads or even those leading the major incident command structure. Regardless, careful consideration should be given to the agency representative who should be fully briefed on the outcomes of the recent intra-agency debriefs. Further debriefing may be required in the context of public or judicial inquiry but in such cases, local or national governments may take a lead role in coordinating.

17.7 Barriers to Debrief

Debrief amongst emergency services addressing major incidents is not uniformly performed. Barriers to its establishment and effective practice differ depending on whether one considers the debrief from a frontline staff or organisational perspective.

Clinical staff concerns include a fear of being criticised or of critiquing colleagues, emotions detracting from the facts, hierarchy preventing junior staff speaking up and lack of participant availability as departmental duties are resumed. These difficulties may be tackled by explaining the critical need of timely debrief to staff and formalising the process through organisational SOPs.

Senior leaders have also identified pre-existing organisational culture, structure, leadership and financial pressures as hindrances to instigating organisational learning processes including debrief [27].

17.8 Format: Hot and Cold Debriefs

Informal debrief will naturally occur between the individuals involved in a major incident immediately after it occurs, but it is important to run a structured debrief in order to guide learning and reflection in an approved format. Without structure, mistakes are missed, good practice is overseen, and valuable information and ideas are not shared.

A common mode of practice is to debrief both immediately after the incident (hot debrief) and a few days to weeks later (cold debrief). There are different hierarchies of cold debrief that are held at local, organisational and multi-agency levels [28, 29].

The purpose of the hot debrief is to incorporate everyone involved in the incident at a time when events are still recent and therefore easy to recall. It also allows an opportunity to "off-load" emotional or traumatic experiences of stressful events that many will not have encountered before. Several hot debriefs may be held simultaneously within an organisation and may be carried out by the separate departments or units involved to highlight any key issues within that unit.

The cold debrief allows a period for reflection and recovery before looking at the incident more objectively. A disadvantage of the cold debrief is that attendance levels are lower due to staffing hours in a shift-based system and the accuracy of the information may be effected as memory of events fade with time.

The key to running an effective debrief is to conduct it in a safe environment that encourages organisational learning and avoids apportioning blame. The following ground rules should be set prior to starting:

1. The purpose of the debrief is to learn.
2. Leave hierarchy at the door.
3. Everyone should contribute, and everyone's contribution should be respected.
4. Contributions should be of what people know, feel and believe.
5. Make no assumptions, be open and honest.
6. Discussing any potential mistakes made should not lead to blame.
7. Everyone will have a different truth to share of the same event.
8. Avoid distractions: No mobile phones.

The basic structure of the debrief asks four questions:

1. What was expected to happen?
2. What actually happened?
3. Was there a difference and why?
4. What can be learned? [28, 30]

An example of how a debrief may be structured is as follows:

1. Introduction
   (a) Overview of the incident
   (b) Reason for the debrief
   (c) Overview of the method of debriefing including the next steps
   (d) Participants introduce themselves and their role in the incident
2. Fact finding
   (a) Document a shared account of the facts and put these in chronological order.
3. What went well? What went badly?
   (a) Participants volunteer an answer for each question and perceived reasons for this
   (b) Discuss how successes can be built upon
   (c) Discuss how failures could be avoided next time
   (d) Discuss what can be done to effect change
4. Summary
   (a) Summarise the discussion
   (b) Identify key learning points

5. Closure
   (a) Questions from participants on any aspects of the response that they are still not clear about
   (b) Give Information on where to seek further help
   (c) Give information on the next stage of the debriefing process [28–30]

17.9 Sharing Lessons Learned from Major Incidents

Despite the increased incidence of major incidents globally, experiences from these events are rarely reported widely. In addition to the various barriers to performing the debrief, in the vast majority of cases, reports formally documenting the lessons learnt, particularly from hot debrief, are marred by poor contemporaneous documentation. Due to the chaotic nature of major incidents, information is often not collected as events occur but instead is recalled hours to weeks after the incident as part of a cold debriefing or reporting process. This can reduce the accuracy of the data collected and contribute to poor reporting. Systems that accommodate the real-time recording of data, particularly passively, could be useful. For example, by using voice recordings, real-time data input electronic applications or global positioning satellite (GPS) data, the need for human participation in data recording and reporting would be minimised whilst maintaining high levels of accuracy.

When they are generated, major incident reports are typically circulated within organisations and when submitted externally, are distributed only at local level. Often reports are difficult to obtain outside of the parent organisation and when accessed are frequently unstructured and unregulated [31].

Though some reports may be found within the grey literature, peer-reviewed journal articles on individual incidents typically take the form of case studies.

These document some experiences but often are difficult to derive useful information from and are hard to compare to other incident reports, preventing useful analysis. There is also publication bias towards those incidents that attract more international attention, particularly from the media [32].

Another factor hindering shared learning from major incidents is the reluctance of organisations to share data for fear of blame or harming institutional reputations. Major incidents are highly politically and socially sensitive, and anxiety over exposing error and vulnerability is understandable. However, for the public and private emergency services involved in the response, the responsibility is not only to those involved in the current major incident but also to those potentially involved in future incidents. Thus, these organisations should be discouraged from withholding information that could improve subsequent responses. The future of major incident reporting must involve the development of a no-blame culture where individual anonymity and a combined effort to learn from mistakes are encouraged.

Whilst there have been several published guidelines on how major incidents and their debriefs ought to be reported, these vary significantly [33]. The crux of the discrepancy relates to which data authors consider to be essential information. Conversely reporting frameworks that are burdened by excessive detail pose an imposition to those attempting to submit reports. There has been a drive in recent times to develop a standardised template for reporting major incidents with agreed definitions and data collection categories which can facilitate comparison and learning across multiple incidents locally, nationally and internationally [34–36]. Recent efforts have also been made to store these standardised reports in a global open access database online, so that lessons can be more readily disseminated [37].

17.10 Conclusions

The key purpose of the debrief is to maximise learning from major incidents. This is paramount given their potential for great harm to human life but relative rarity. Debrief optimises operational capability ahead of the next event through adaptations of any existing major incident plans and in some instances leads to the creation of new recommendations.

This process needs to be carried out in a timely fashion and at multiple organisational levels to capture both frontline and incident command staff experiences, as well as experiences amongst different agencies. No response to unexpected mass casualty events is flawless and there are always improvements to be made, but these are best achieved through a constructive and open approach.

The debrief represents a fundamental part of the learning process around these grave events and is augmented through interdisciplinary and cross-border sharing of learning outcomes.

17.11 Key Recommendations

Before debrief session

1. *Ensure that debriefs are incorporated into institutional major incident plans, including templates clarifying format and points to be covered.*
2. *Brief staff early on within a major incident regarding when debriefs are expected to take place to ensure maximum attendance.*
3. *During protracted incidents, make arrangements for early preliminary hot debriefs at times of staff changeover.*

During debrief session

4. *Use a trained facilitator who understands how to conduct debrief safely and appropriately in the context of an emotionally difficult situation.*
5. *Follow a planned format from either local SOPs or other guidelines to ensure that a full range of points are covered.*
6. *Employ an open no-blame approach to the debrief, with all participants encouraged to contribute constructively.*
7. *Practise emotional first aid through exercising compassion and support, addressing welfare needs and not attempting to tackle emotional trauma directly. Where concerns arise, colleagues can be referred to mental health professionals at a later stage.*

8. *Record the discussions contemporaneously and where feasible use digital recording devices and upload to secure central storage platforms to reduce loss of data and reduce additional workload.*
9. *Ensure that debriefs occur with the appropriate personnel at appropriate times: hot debriefs amongst smaller teams working together at the time of the incident, cold debrief in the follow-up to the incident at organisational level with key personnel and representatives from smaller teams. Consider inter-agency debriefs further down the line.*

After debrief session

10. *Create a well-structured debrief report using local or publically available guidelines on report format.*
11. *In addition to any mandated submissions of reports within the organisation, where possible share the report or key findings with other agencies locally and with organisations nationally and internationally (consider majorincidentreporting.net).*
12. *Consider the lessons learnt both from local events, other agencies and from international reports to make timely changes to organisational systems and augment major incident plans.*

References

1. Leaning J, Guha-Sapir D. Natural disasters, armed conflict and public health. N Engl J Med. 2013;369:1836–42.
2. Global Terrorism Index 2017. Institute for Economics and Peace. 2017. http://visionofhumanity.org/app/uploads/2017/11/Global-Terrorism-Index-2017.pdf. Accessed 15 Feb 2018.
3. Blom L, Black JM. Major incidents. BMJ. 2014;28:348.
4. Mackway-Jones K. Major incident medical management: the practical approach at the scene. 3rd ed. Chichester: Blackwell-Wiley; 2012.
5. Kolb D. Experiential learning: experience as the source of learning and development. 1st ed. Englewood Cliffs: Prentice Hall; 1984.
6. Hecker A. Knowledge beyond the individual? Making sense of a notion of collective knowledge in organization theory. Organ Stud. 2012;33:423–45.
7. Rajan A, Lank E, Chappel K. Good practices in knowledge creation and exchange. 1st ed. Tunbridge Wells: Create; 1998.
8. Easterby-Smith M, Araujo L. Organizational learning: current debates and opportunities. In: Easterby-Smith M, Araujo L, Burgoyne J, editors. Organizational learning and the learning organization: developments in theory and practice. London: Sage; 1999. p. 1–21.
9. Collison C, Parcell G. Learning to fly: practical knowledge management from leading and learning organisations. Chichester: Capstone Press; 2004.
10. Vashdi DR, Bamberger PA, Erez M, Weiss-Meilik A. Briefing-debriefing: using a reflexive organizational learning model from the military to enhance the performance of surgical teams. Hum Resour Manage. 2007;46:115–42.
11. Wiltshire Policeforce Procedure. Debriefing procedure (critical incidents). 2017. http://www.wiltshire.police.uk/media/329/Critical-Incident-Debrief-Procedure/pdf/Critical_Incident_Debrief_Procedure.pdf. Accessed 15 Feb 2018.

12. Marcellin JD. The Pilot Factor: a new look into CRM. Dayton: Plane & Simple Solutions; 2014.
13. National Health Service, England. Human factors in healthcare: a concordat from the National Quality Board. 2013. https://www.england.nhs.uk/wp-content/uploads/2013/11/nqb-hum-fact-concord.pdf. Accessed 15 Feb 2018.
14. Catchpole K. Spreading human factors expertise in healthcare: untangling the knots in people and systems. BMJ Qual Saf. 2013;22:793–7.
15. Tannenbaum SI, Cerasoli CP. Do team and individual debriefs enhance performance? A meta-analysis. Hum Factors. 2013;55:231–45.
16. Association of Anaesthetists of Great Britain and Ireland. Catastrophes in anaesthetic practice – dealing with the aftermath. 2005. https://www.aagbi.org/sites/default/files/catastrophes05.pdf. Accessed 15 Feb 2018.
17. Shalev AY. Post traumatic stress disorder. Prim Psychiatry. 2001;8:41–6.
18. Hunt P, Greaves I. Oxford manual of major incident management. Oxford: Oxford University Press; 2017.
19. Williams R, Bisson J, Ajdukovic D, Kemp V, Olff M, Alexander D, Hacker Hughtes J, Bevan P. Guidance for responding to the psychosocial and mental health needs of people affected by disasters or major incidents. 2009. . http://www.healthplanning.co.uk/nato. Accessed 15 Feb 2018.
20. Lederman L. Debriefing: a critical re-examination of the post-experience analytic process with implications for its effective use. Simul Games. 1984;15:415–31.
21. Rose SC, Bisson J, Churchill R, Wessely S. Psychological debriefing for preventing post traumatic stress disorder (PTSD). Cochrane Database Syst Rev. 2002;(2):CD000560. https://doi.org/10.1002/14651858.CD000560.
22. Hawker DM, Durkin J, Hawker DS. To debrief or not to debrief our heroes: that is the question. Clin Psychol Psychother. 2011;18:453–63.
23. Everly G, Lating J. The Johns Hopkins guide to psychological first aid. Baltimore: John Hopkins University Press; 2017.
24. The Task Force on International Trauma Training of ISTSS. Guidelines for international training in mental health and psychosocial interventions for trauma exposed populations in clinical and community settings. https://www.istss.org/ISTSS_Main/media/Documents/ISTSS_guidelines_for_training.pdf. Accessed 15 Feb 2018.
25. College of Policing. Operations: briefing and debriefing. 2013. https://www.app.college.police.uk/app-content/operations/briefing-and-debriefing/. Accessed 15 Feb 2018.
26. "debrief, n.1". Oxford dictionaries online. 2018. Oxford University Press. https://en.oxforddictionaries.com/definition/debrief Accessed 15 Feb 2018.
27. McLelland J. Organisational learning and how marginal gains can be made by debriefing and improving how they do activities next time, making best use of knowledge and management. 2015. http://library.college.police.uk/docs/theses/MCLELLAND-organisational-learning-2015.docx. Accessed 15 Feb 2018.
28. NHS England. NHS England Emergency Preparedness, Resilience and Response (EPRR) Business Continuity Management toolkit; 2016.
29. Norman S. Organisational debriefing and reporting. In: Norman S, et al., editors. Health emergency planning: a handbook for practitioners. London: TSO; 2006. p. 121–5.
30. Campbell M, Miller K, McNicholas K. Post event debriefs: a commitment to learning how to better care for patients and staff. Jt Comm J Qual Patient Saf. 2016;42(1):41–7.
31. Carley S, Mackway-Jones K, Donnan S. Major incidents in Britain over the past 28 years: the case for the centralised reporting of major incidents. J Epidemiol Community Health. 1998;52:392–8.
32. Smith E, Wasiak J, Sen A, Archer F, Burke F. Three decades of disaster: a review of disaster specific literature from 1977-2009. Prehosp Disaster Med. 2009;24:306–11.
33. Fattah S, Rehn M, Wisborg T. Implementing a template for major incident reporting: experiences from the first year. Scand J Trauma Resusc Emerg Med. 2015;23:55.

34. Bradt D, Aitken P. Disaster medicine reporting: the need for new guidelines and the CONFIDE statement. Emerg Med Australas. 2010;22:483–7.
35. World Association for Disaster and Emergency Medicine & Nordic Society for Disaster Medicine. Health disaster management: guidelines for evaluation and research in the "Utstein style". Prehosp Disaster Med. 2003;17(Suppl):1–167.
36. Hardy S, Fattah S. Trials and tribulations: how we established a major incident database. Scand J Trauma Resusc Emerg Med. 2017;5:7.
37. Major Incident Reporting. http://majorincidentreporting.net. Accessed 15 Feb 2018.
38. Hardy S. Major incidents in England. BMJ. 2015;31:350.

Ethics in Mass Casualty Incidents

18

Boris E. Sakakushev

Ethics implications are at the core of preparation, policies, response, and recovery of MCI.

In order to understand more clearly the close relation of ethics and disasters, we have to answer three basic questions:

1. Why do we need to know the ethical basis of disaster preparation and response?
2. What is special about disasters that motivates people to act and respond ethically and how is this manifested?
3. What are the relevant ethical principles that form the basis of our actions and reactions?

There are three aspects of a disaster on man—physical, emotional, and spiritual. The specific mental health stressors are self or family member injury, life threat fear and panic during event, relocation, peri-traumatic responses, and horror separation from family and property damage or financial loss.

Persons with disabilities may experience personal vulnerability as well as protective factors. They may suffer systemic vulnerability or protective factors across environments and ecologies. Disaster response practices intend to diminish risk factors.

What is special about disasters that motivates people to act and respond ethically?

Ethics contains basic human values of compassion, empathy, respect for dignity of others, and professional codes of conduct.

Ethics is important and versatile and currently is very relevant to society because it includes social responsibility and requires governance.

B. E. Sakakushev (✉)
General Surgery Department, University of Medicine Plovdiv, University Hospital St George, Plovdiv, Bulgaria

Y. Kluger et al. (eds.), *WSES Handbook of Mass Casualties Incidents Management*, Hot Topics in Acute Care Surgery and Trauma,
https://doi.org/10.1007/978-3-319-92345-1_18

The roots of ethics relevance date from Ancient Greece "Do good work consider end use" (Aristotle) and Renaissance: "Evaluate both ends and means" (Kant) and are updated to plan holistically by the systems theory, contributing to knowledge.

The definition of ethics or the moral philosophy summarizing several definitions is "determining rights and wrongs, selecting actions to achieve good results, evaluating motives." Ethics is "the achievement of wisdom, choosing actions that are beneficial and acceptable long term or sustainable" [1].

"Ethics is not about what is—but what should be."

The basic theories and principles of ethics are ethical relativism: morality varies between people and societies according to their cultural norms and universal or objective moral theories: fundamental principles that are invariant throughout time and space [2].

The four "types" of ethics are:

1. Metaethics (what is good?)
2. Normative ethics (what should we do?)
3. Applied ethics (ethics in work and lives?)
4. Descriptive ethics (morals people follow)

Codes of ethics is the applying of ethics to a profession or discipline like engineering, medicine, law, journalism, psychology, etc.

The golden rule of symmetrical ethics is do to others what you want them to do to you, as well as, if you demand from others, demand from yourself (even more). The idea is to see yourself as the others, or transmitting empathy.

Asymmetrical ethics is when one party has more resources, knowledge, and power. Ethics compliance is applied in laws, standards, guidelines, and morals, where the "compliance officer" has to "follow standard". This ensures, that though difficult, response organization does not go wrong [3]. Positive ethics is when it is contributing positively to society organization, profession or environment. According to Aristotle (384–322) (Fig. 18.1), the moralist states: my life view is superior; other views are inferior; I have the answers; I need no other authority. The ethicist claims: my life view is based on reflection; I evaluate life views; I have questions; I respect oath.

The basic principles of ethics are openness and privacy. Openness means to publish, register, compare, analyze, and find missing information, while privacy includes personal room integrity, harmful, embarrassmental, wrong or wrongly used information.

Ethical principles applied during MCI should be based on humanitarian assistance, information and participation during disasters, compulsory evacuation of populations, respect of dignity and persons, emergency assistance for the most vulnerable persons, measures to safeguard and rehabilitate the environment, strengthening resilience to the effects of disasters, protection of economic, social, cultural, civil and political rights [4].

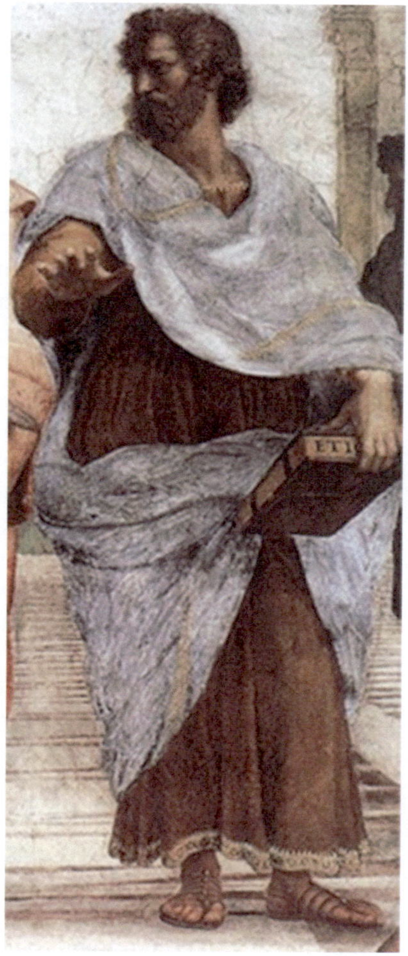

Fig. 18.1 Aristotle (384–322)

The relevant ethical principles are substantive and procedural. The substantive principles are individual liberty, protection of the public from harm, proportionality and reciprocity, privacy, duty to provide care, equity and solidarity, trust and stewardship. The procedural principles are reasonability, openness and transparency, inclusiveness, responsiveness, and accountability [5].

Disaster ethics is addressed in three phases [6]:

- Pre-disaster (pre-event) or preventive phase
- Disaster (event/crisis) and early response phase
- Post-disaster (post-event) or rehabilitation phase

The disaster ethics in the early response phase are those of non-maleficence, beneficence, justice, and the respect for autonomy. Reaching the disaster site as quickly as possible is the most crucial step. "Public health institutions should act in a timely manner on the information they have within the resources and the mandate given to them by the public" [7].

In the early response phase—the triage, as the second most important step, is considered as critical in the distribution of limited medical resources, where highest priority should be given to the principles of beneficence and justice. The mass casualty approach follows the principle of decision-making for saving more lives. It is the "triage" principle, not life support.

World Medical Association statement on medical ethics in the event of disasters says that in selecting the patients, the physician should consider only their medical status, and should exclude any other consideration based on non-medical criteria [8]. Triage and ethics in MCI unite on saving more lives, where selecting and referring only the "red" coded patients is a rule without exceptions, which has proved its effectiveness through practice and research. In disaster medicine management, one must follow not only principles of triage, life support, and on time emergency treatment, but also go along with ethical issues. It is exactly like in surgery teaching and learning—acquiring and implementing knowledge, skills, and attitudes. Discussions on triage decisions with respect to the victim's age, gender, social status, ethnic origin, or profession (e.g., health workers) also conflict with the basic right to live at the individual level and justice principle, in general. "Ideological issues must not eclipse the humanistic priorities embodied in ethical rules" [9]. Practically, having 20 critically ill victims at open field, one have to "triage" all of them as fast as possible (15–20 s), giving them chance for life. One even may become unlikable, speak loud, cry to hear you, or obey orders. Here ethical issues are not obligatory—one does not choose children, pregnant, or disabled. All have the priority of the "red" code. The first one is the closest one. The second is next to him. One cannot afford spending time on observing all the 20 injured. There are reasons for excluding disabled in algorithms:

- Individuals will need resources for prolonged period of use.
- They are deemed to have a poor quality of life post-treatment.
- They have a limited long-term prognosis as a result of their disabilities.

Triage is a form of rationing care delivery. Rationing delivery of care is justified only in situations in which the amount of resources available is less than "adequate" (first and foremost, insufficient to meet the critical requirements) [10].

The traditional "transvertical" triage advocates with scarce resources to provide the maximum benefit to the population, even if it means that individual victims that can be saved under other circumstances are sacrificed for the greater good. The "longitudinal" triage necessitates sacrificing victims now, for the benefit of future victims. In mass casualty medicine, the clinical paradigm is replaced by the rescue paradigm in which it is necessary to save lives and minimize aggregate morbidity [11].

Questions of where consideration for the individual ends and the rights of the majority begin remain valid ones in the face of limited resources [12].

Triage decisions must not discriminate against terrorists, despite the highly emotional situation in which attackers and victims are treated simultaneously on-site [13].

Defining specified standards prior to the emergency response will methodologically enable improvement of the successful response to different types of emergency scenarios, regardless of their variable components [14, 15].

In light of the importance for expanding the science of disaster management, the complexity of acquiring informed consent while conducting studies in the realm of disaster medicine should be widely reviewed and weighed [16].

For daily triage decisions, a new model of resource allocation, known as accountability for reasonableness, claims that resource allocation should proceed on the basis of relevant criteria, that are public, that decision-making be accountable, and that an appeal process exists in cases of conflict [17]. Healthcare organizations can deploy a triage and scarce resource allocation team to oversee and guide ethically challenging clinical decision-making during a crisis period. The goal is to help healthcare organizations and clinicians balance public health responsibilities and their duty to individual patients during emergencies in as equitable and humane a manner as possible [18]. To understand whether disaster triage, as currently advocated and practiced in the western world, is actually ethical, we should clarify whether resources truly are limited, whether specific numbers should dictate disaster response, and whether triage decisions should be based on age or social worth [19, 20].

People affected by a disaster may not be capable of responding to human rights violations, so it is the first responders who must be cognizant of their responsibility to protect the victims' dignity and rights. Ethical treatment of survivors entails a crucial blend of knowledge about ethnic culture, religious beliefs, and human rights. A strong awareness of ethical principles is merely a beginning step to well-informed decision-making in disaster situations [21].

Research ethics should take the format of an iterative evolving and constructive learning process, with a time of reflection and critical debate [22]. Potential need for non-standard ethics review procedures for MCI settings is to ensure appropriate dissemination of disaster research results among researchers, to share information, and develop projects to evaluate how well the ethical issues are addressed in the research. Particular attention should be given to assessing participants' perceptions of how ethics is addressed in specific projects [23].

The Social Contract states: "Government has an obligation, to prepare citizens for survival in second states of nature caused by disaster. Such preparation requires implementation through public policy." (John Locke). These rights are presumed in the US Declaration of Independence and protected by the first ten amendments of the constitution [24].

Throughout the centuries there are many local and national (Figs. 18.2 and 18.3) as well as global (Fig. 18.4) documents which can be related to ethics in MCI.

Professional codes of ethics act as: "Professions governed by codes of ethics approved by their members function on the assumption that these codes will not be violated in practice" [24].

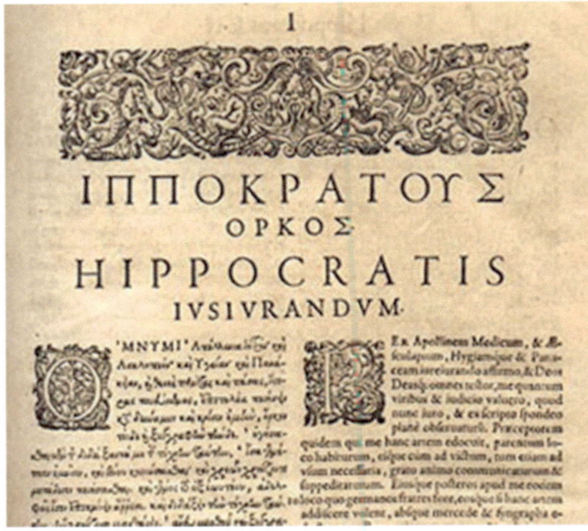

Fig. 18.2 Oath of Hippocrates 4c B.C.

1. Oath of Hippocrates 4th century B.C.E.
2. Oath of Initiation
3. Oath of Asaph
4. Advice to Physician
5. 17 Rule of Enjuin
6. Five Commandments and Ten Requirements 1617
7. A Physician's Ethical Duties from Kholasah al Hekman
8. Daily Prayer of a Physician (prayer of Moses Maimonidies) 1793
9. Code of Ethics AMA 1847
10. Declaration of Geneva, WMA 1948
11. Intl Code of Medical Ethics 1949
12. Principles of Medical Ethics AMA 1957
13. Oath of Soviet Physicians 1971
14. Oath of a Muslim Physician, Islamic Medical Assoc. of North America 1977
15. Islamic Code of Medical Ethics, Kuwait Document, Islamic Organization for Medical Sciences 1981
16. Regulations on Criteria for Medical Ethics and their Implementation – China –1988
17. Health Care Ethics Guide, Catholic Health Assoc. of Canada 1991
18. Solemn Oath of a Physician of Russia 1992
19. Code of Ethics, AmericanOsteopathic Assn 1998
20. Code of Ethics and Guide to Ethical Behaviour of physicians.
21. Canadian Medical Association1996
22. Code of Ethics Chile –1983
23. Code of Ethics Brazil -1988
24. Code of Ethics Norway –2000
25. Code of Ethics Japan 1991
26. Ethical and Religious Directives for Catholic Health Facilities 1971, rev. 2001
27. Declaration of Prof. Responsibility AMA2001
28. Charter on Medical Professionalism (2002)
29. New Zealand Medical Assoc. 2002

Fig. 18.3 "Ethical Directives for the Practice of Medicine" from fourth century B.C.E till 21st c. [25]

1. Human Rights first declared internationally in 1948 in the United Nations'(UN's) Declaration of Human Rights. Not an international law – global paradigm
2. United Nations Charter earth for All in the 21st Century" World Health Organization (WHO)
3. 1985 Tokyo Declaration by the World Medical Association against physicians being involved in torture
4. 1988 United Nations Resolution, the "Right to Intervene"
5. International Humanitarian Law (IHL-comprises the Geneva Conventions and the Hague Conventions)
6. The Helsinki Declaration protects the patients' rights and integrity with regard to research. Ethics Landmark but not practical for disaster, endorsed at the General Assembly of the World Medical Association in Helsinki, Finland in 1964

Fig. 18.4 Global ethics documents relevant to ethics in MCI are [26]

Biohazards can be considered in certain circumstances as MCI. Therefore, exportation of hazards constitutes both ethical and legal issues. Solidarity requires "deliberate and freely chosen unity among certain groups or populations." "When referring to healthcare, solidarity means the obligation to share the financial risks of illness and handicap with others not necessarily of one's own social group." Joint responsibility constitutes the shared responsibility between governments, communities, businesses, and individuals. Civil laws must assure non-discrimination principles of the law, which require equal access and prohibit discrimination against people with disabilities in all aspects of emergency planning, response, and recovery [27].

The principles of internal displacement adopted by the United Nations Commission and the General Assembly are aimed to protect all internally displaced persons in internal conflict situations, natural disasters, and other situations of forced displacement. The principle of impartiality states: "It makes no discrimination based upon nationality, race, religious beliefs, class, or political opinions."

The American Red Cross, as a member of the International Red Cross and Red Crescent Movement, adheres to the fundamental principles of the International Red Cross and Red Crescent Movement [28]. The code of conduct for International Red Cross and Red Crescent Movement and NGOs in disaster relief was drawn up in 1992 by the Steering Committee for Humanitarian Response (SCHR) to set ethical standards for organizations involved in humanitarian work [29]. In 1994, the SCHR adopted the code and made the signing of it a condition for membership in the alliance. "The cardinal virtues of disaster response are prudence, courage, justice, stewardship, vigilance, self-effacing charity, and communication."

The standard of care is a case- and time-specific analytical process in medical decision-making, reflecting a clinical benchmark of acceptable quality medical care [30]. Professional ethics is the accepted principles or moral codes that conforms to the accepted standards of that profession [31].

Disasters vary considerably with respect to their time, place, and extent; therefore, ethical questions may not always have "one-size-fits-all" answers. On the other hand, embedding ethical values and principles in every aspect of healthcare is of vital importance. Reviewing legal and organizational regulations, developing healthcare related guidelines, and disaster recovery plans, establishing on-call ethics committees, as well as adequate in-service training of healthcare workers for ethical competence are among the most critical steps. It is only by making efforts before disasters, that ethical challenges can be minimized in disaster responses [32]. The Japan disaster mental health guidelines provide a comprehensive description on what to do and say in times of disaster. With dissemination and use of guidelines, local mental health systems can be improved and will be better prepared ahead of future disasters [33]. The Delphi technique can be used for reaching consensus of data, comprising process, structure and outcome indicators, identified as essential for recording indicators essential for data reporting from the response of major incidents. It can serve as a basis for a generally acceptable national register [34].

Ethical principles applied prior to disaster are prevention measures, good quality healthy environment, education, training and awareness, participation—public input at national and local level, freedom of expression, and access to justice [4]. Ethical approach to allocation of scarce resources and triage should be based on fairness, transparency, consistency, proportionality, accountability, and a duty to attempt to obtain best outcome for the greatest number of patients with available resources—it does not mean to save the most lives, because a comfortable death may be a good outcome (Fig. 18.5) [35]. Ethical dilemmas and codes of conduct in MCI include announcing bad news under pressure to patient (if conscious), to relatives, friends and to media (Fig. 18.6).

Responsible for ethical information in disasters are the local emergency management command centers, including police, fire, EMS, public health agencies and departments, bioethics committees, physician, and nursing education teams. The leader in MCI acting under pressure must address the team in brief, precise, encouraging, positive, and definite manner.

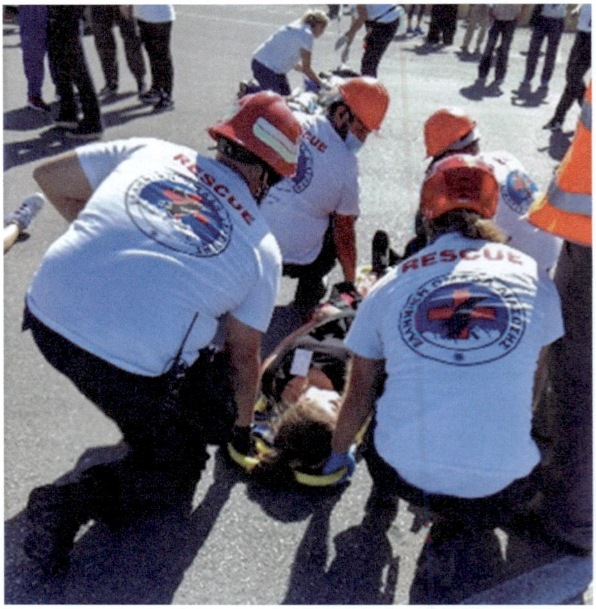

Fig. 18.5 Ethical approach in triage

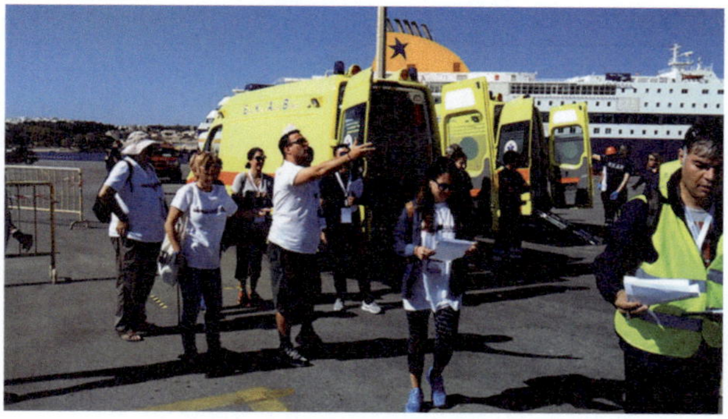

Fig. 18.6 Announcing bad news to relatives

The code of professional ethics for rehabilitation counselors contains primary responsibility, proper diagnosis of mental disorders, respect for confidentiality and adapting to work environment. They should maintain roles and relationships, appropriate termination, referral and transfer of services based on competences like preparation and response, cultural diversity, advocacy and accessibility, scientific bases for intervention, technique/procedure/modalities skills and finally yet importantly—monitor effectiveness. Strategies to maximize care concern space, structure, medications and staff. Common activities are put patient beds in hallways, conference rooms, tents, use operating rooms only for urgent cases, supply/sterilize and reuse disposable equipment, limit drugs/vaccines/ventilators to patients most likely to benefit, prioritize comfort care for patients who will die/ and have family members help with feeding and other basic patient tasks.

The future objectives before ethics in MCI are:

- Encourage and consolidate knowledge networks
- Mobilize and train disaster volunteers—army, police firemen, scouts and guides, civil defense, guards
- Build capacity and learn from best practices

The future directions are:

- Anticipatory governance—simulation exercises, and scenario analysis
- Knowledge systems and coping practices
- Living with risk—community-based disaster risk management
- Inclusive, participatory, gender sensitive, child friendly, eco-friendly and disabled friendly disaster management
- Technology driven but people owned
- Knowledge management—documentation and dissemination of good practices
- Public private partnership

What to expect? A killer asteroid, coronal mass sun ejection (Fig. 18.7), a massive quake, thermohaline circulation shutting down, global pandemic (Fig. 18.8), wrong genetic manipulation etc.?

Why do so many major world disasters happen on the 26th? Is “26” the new “13” (Fig. 18.9).

The challenge of disaster preparedness is how we give the best care possible under the worst possible circumstances.

Investments in preparedness and prevention (mitigation) will yield sustainable results, rather than spending money on relief after a disaster because most disasters are predictable, especially in their seasonality and the disaster-prone areas, which are vulnerable.

The future directions in meeting goals in legislation and recommendations are developing ethical guidelines. These require legislative task force, state committee, ethics board, studies and regulations with resolutions and considerations. The considerations for developing ethical guidelines comprise of resource owner, recognizable voice, big city and budget disaster allocation, public and research activities like discussions, presentations and conferences, ethics research and analysis center, and state agencies.

Education and training are especially important in [36]:

- Disaster planning and rehearsal
- Integration of local, regional, and national resources into a disaster system
- Hospital emergency incident command systems (HEICS)
- Communications and security
- Media relations
- Protection of healthcare delivery personnel and facilities
- Detection and decontamination of biological, chemical, and radiation exposure
- Triage principles and implementation
- Logistics of medical evaluation, stabilization, disposition, and treatment of victims
- Record-keeping and post-disaster debriefing, critique, and reporting

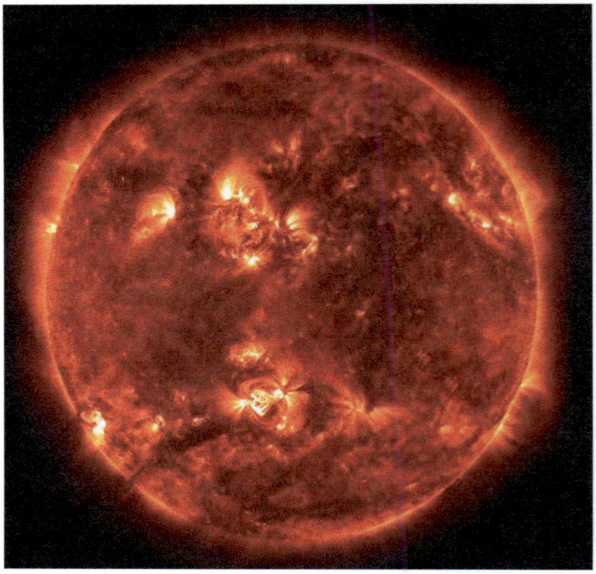

Fig. 18.7 A coronal mass ejection can cause power outages and starvation

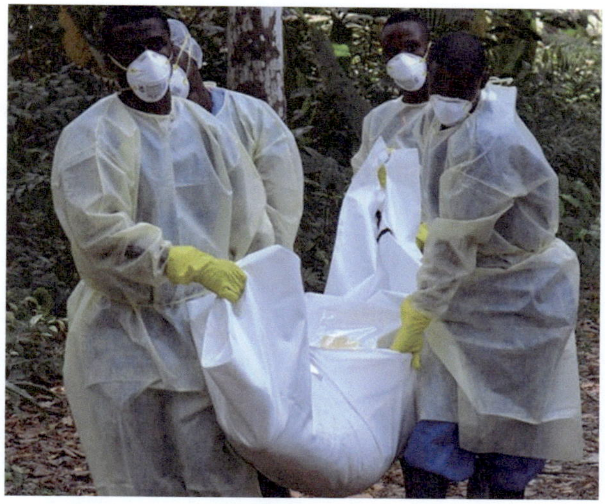

Fig. 18.8 Major solar storm 2015–2025

Fig. 18.9 The curse of 26th

1. North America earthquake 26 Jan 1700
2. Krakatau volcano 26 Aug 1883 (36,000 dead)
3. The Rhodes earthquake 26 June 1926
4. Kansu,China earthquake 26 Dec 1932 (70,000 d)
5. Turkey earthquke 26 Dec 1939 (41,000 dead)
6. Portugal earthquake 26 Jan 1951 (30,000 dead)
7. Yugoslavia earthquake 26 July 1963
8. China Earthquake 26 July 1976
9. Sabah Tidal waves 26 Dec 1996 (1,000 dead)
10. Gujrat Earthquake 26 January 2001
11. Bam, Iran earthquake 26 Dec 2003 (60,000 d)
12. Tsunami in Indian Ocean 26th Dec 2004
13. Aceh Tsunami 26 Dec 2004
14. Mumbai floods 26 July 2005
15. Tasik earthquake 26 June 2010
16. Taiwan earthquake 26 July 2010
17. Mentawai Tsunami 26 October 2010
18. Merapi volcanic eruption 26 Oct 2010
19. Japan Earthquake 26 Feb 2010
20. Nepal Earthquake 26 April 2015
21. Hindukush Afghan Earthquake 26 Oct 2015

- Critical incident stress management (CISM)
- Published research and experience in disaster management

Strategic international partnership is required to collaboratively share the risks and strengthen societal resilience towards MCI. Regional and global cooperation have to be developed to enhance preparedness to deal with large-scale hazards and mitigate sustainability, protection and empowerment, and recovery and rehabilitation programs based on the best and most robust scientific information and coordinated public programs in urban and rural areas [37].

In MCI, specific knowledge, skills, training, and teamwork are necessary to face the ethical dilemmas and implement the appropriate codes of conduct alongside with some simple moral human concerns like honesty, sincerity, sympathy, and trust (Fig. 18.10).

> "A physician's life is a constant and losing battle against obsolescence." Mark M. Ravitch, 1910–1989 (Fig. 18.11).

Fig. 18.10 Teamwork in MCI

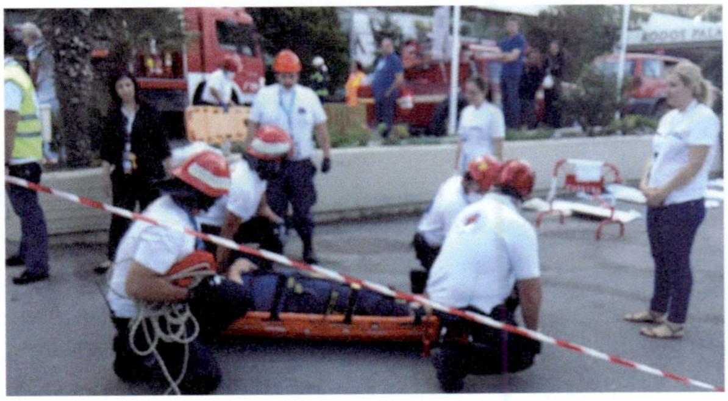

Fig. 18.11 Mark M. Ravitch, 191

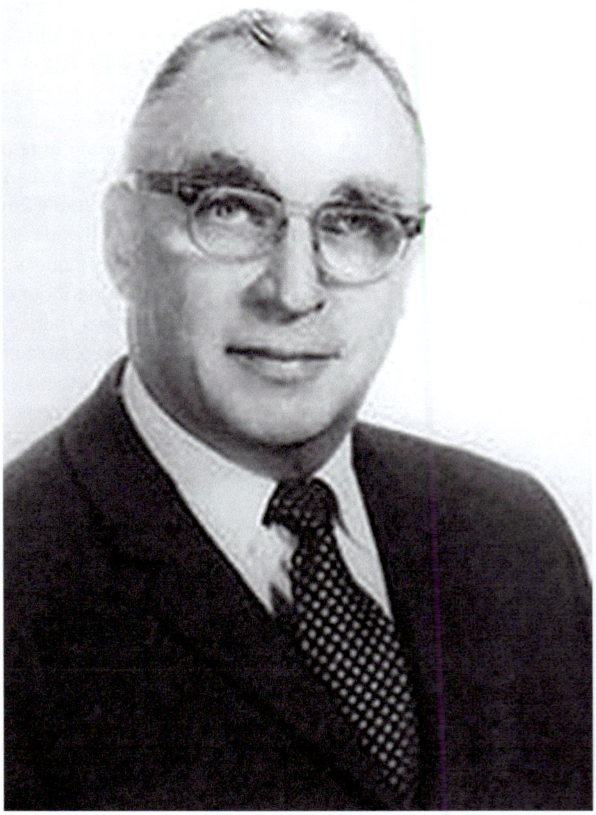

References

1. Sternberg J, editor. Wisdom: its nature, origins, and development. Cambridge: Cambridge University Press; 2003. ISBN10 0521367182.
2. Etkin D, Davis I. The search for principles of disaster management. Working draft paper, 30 May 2007, 28p. Forms of Ethics.
3. The Ethics & Compliance Officer Association (ECOA). December 2010. www.theecoa.org.
4. Prieur M. Ethical principles on disaster risk reduction and people's resilience. European and Mediterranean Major Hazards Agreement (EUR-OPA). 2012. http://www.coe.int/t/dg4/majorhazards/ressources/pub/Ethical-Principles-Publication_EN.pdf.
5. Ross U, et al. Stand on guard for thee. Ethical considerations in preparedness planning for pandemic influenza. A report of the University of Toronto Joint Centre for Bioethics Pandemic Influenza Working Group; 2005.
6. Karadag C, Hakan A. Ethical dilemmas in disaster medicine. Iran Red Crescent Med J. 2012;14(10):1–11.
7. Principles of the ethical practice of public health, Version 2.2 © 2002. Public Health Leadership Society.
8. World Medical Association. Statement on medical ethics in the event of disasters. Updated version. South Africa: WMA General Assembly. 2006. http://www.wma.net/en/30publications/10policies/d7/index.html/.
9. Halpern P, Larkin G. Ethical issues in the provision of emergency medical care in multiple casualty incidents and disasters. In: Ciottone G, editor. Disaster medicine. 3rd ed. Philedelphia: Elsevier Mosby; 2006.
10. Domres B, Koch M, Manger A, Becker H. Ethics and triage. Prehosp Disaster Med. 2001;16(1):53–8.
11. Singh S. Book review of "The Ethics of Coercion in Mass Casualty Medicine" by Griffin Trotter MD, PhD. Philos Ethics Humanit Med. 2007;2(1):20.
12. Hawryluck L. Ethics review: position papers and policies – are they really helpful to front-line ICU teams? Crit Care. 2006;10(6):242.
13. Adini B, Ohana A, Furman E, Ringel R, Golan Y, Fleshler E, Keren U, Reisner S. Learning lessons in emergency management: the 4th international conference on healthcare system preparedness and response to emergencies and disasters. Disaster Mil Med. 2016;2(1):16.
14. Leaning J, Guha-Sapir D. Natural disasters, armed conflict, and public health. N Engl J Med. 2013;369:1836–42.
15. Gardemann J, Wilp T. The Humanitarian Charter and minimum standards in humanitarian response are applicable in German refugee facilities. Bundesgesundheitsblatt Gesundheitsforschung Gesundheitsschutz. 2016;59(5):556–60.
16. Frith L, Appleton R, Iyer A, Messahel S, Hickey H, Gamble C. Doing challenging research studies in a patient-centred way: a qualitative study to inform a randomized controlled trial in the paediatric emergency care setting. BMJ Open. 2014;4:e0050.
17. Daniels N, Sabin J. Setting limits fairly: can we learn to share medical resources? Oxford: Oxford University Press.
18. Kuschner W, Pollard J, Ezeji-Okoye S. Ethical triage and scarce resource allocation during public health emergencies: tenets and procedures. Hosp Top. 2007;85(3):16–25.
19. Sztajnkrycer M, Madsen B, Alejandro Báez A. Unstable ethical plateaus and disaster triage. Emerg Med Clin North Am. 2006;24(3):749–68.
20. Holt G. Making difficult ethical decisions in patient care during natural disasters and other mass casualty events. Otolaryngol Head Neck Surg. 2008;139(2):181–6.
21. Varghese S. Cultural, ethical, and spiritual implications of natural disasters from the survivors' perspective. Crit Care Nurs Clin North Am. 2010;22(4):515–22.
22. Schopper D, Dawson A, Upshur R, Ahmad A, Jesani A, Ravinetto R, Segelid M, Sheel S, Singh J. Innovations in research ethics governance in humanitarian settings. BMC Med Ethics. 2015;16:10.
23. Mezinska S, Kakuk P, Mijaljica G, Waligóra M, O'Mathúna D. Research in disaster settings: a systematic qualitative review of ethical guidelines. BMC Med Ethics. 2016;17:1.

24. Zack N. Ethics for disaster. Series: studies in social, political, and legal philosophy. Lanham: Maryland Rowman & Littlefield Publishers; 2009.
25. The Hippocratic Oath: text, translation, and interpretation, by Ludwig Edelstein. Baltimore: Johns Hopkins Press, 1943.
26. Health Disaster Management Guidelines for Evaluation and Research in the Utstein Style Chapter 8: Ethical issues. Prehosp Disast Med. 2002;17(Suppl 3):128–143.
27. FEMA. http://www.fema.gov/iv-non-dscrimination-principles-law.
28. Steering Committee for Humanitarian Response. http://www.redcross.org/portal/site/en/menuitem.d229a5f06620c6052b1ecfbf43181aa0/?vgnextoid=f5195032f953e110VgnVCM10000089f0870aRCRD&vgnextchannel=d18859f392ce8110VgnVCM10000030f3870aRCRD; http://en.wikipedia.org/wiki/.
29. Steering Committee for Humanitarian Response. http://en.wikipedia.org/wiki/.
30. American College of Medical Quality, policy 3. http://www.acmq.org/policies/policies3and4.pdf/.
31. Geale SK. The ethics of disaster management. Disaster Prev Manage. 2012;21(4):445–62.
32. Karadag C, Hakan K. Ethical dilemmas in disaster medicine. Iran Red Crescent Med J. 2012;14(10):602–12.
33. Suzuki Y, Fukasawa M, Nakajima S, Narisawa T, Kim Y. Development of disaster mental health guidelines through the Delphi process in Japan. Int J Mental Health Syst. 2012;6(1):7.
34. Rådestad M, Jirwe M, Castrén M, Svensson L, Gryth D, Rüter A. Essential key indicators for disaster medical response suggested to be included in a national uniform protocol for documentation of major incidents: a Delphi study. Scand J Trauma Resusc Emerg Med. 2013;21(1):68.
35. Hick J, Hanfling D, Cantrill S. Allocating scarce resources in disasters: emergency department principles. Ann Emerg Med. 2012;59(3):177–87.
36. Statement on disaster and mass casualty management. The following statement was developed by the College's Ad Hoc Committee on Disaster and Mass Casualty Management of the Committee on Trauma, and was approved by the Board of Regents at its June 2003 meeting.
37. Tambo E. Non-conventional humanitarian interventions on Ebola outbreak crisis in West Africa: health, ethics and legal implications. Infect Dis Poverty. 2014;3(1):42.

MIX
Papier aus verantwortungsvollen Quellen
Paper from responsible sources
FSC® C105338

If you have any concerns about our products,
you can contact us on
ProductSafety@springernature.com

In case Publisher is established outside the EU,
the EU authorized representative is:
Springer Nature Customer Service Center GmbH
Europaplatz 3, 69115 Heidelberg, Germany

Printed by Libri Plureos GmbH
in Hamburg, Germany